A PRACTICAL APPROACH
TO THE MANAGEMENT OF SALIVA

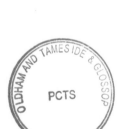

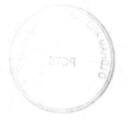

A PRACTICAL APPROACH TO THE MANAGEMENT OF SALIVA

SECOND EDITION

Amanda Scott
and
Hilary Johnson

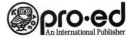

8700 Shoal Creek Boulevard
Austin, Texas 78757-6897
800/897-3202   Fax 800/397-7633
www.proedinc.com

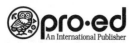

© 1993, 2004 by PRO-ED, Inc.
8700 Shoal Creek Boulevard
Austin, Texas 78757-6897
800/897-3202   Fax 800/397-7633
www.proedinc.com

Library of Congress Cataloging-in-Publication Data

Scott, Amanda, B.App.Sci.
  A practical approach to the management of saliva / Amanda Scott and Hilary Johnson.—
2nd ed.
    p. ; cm.
  Rev. ed. of: A practical approach to saliva control / by Hilary Johnson and Amanda
Scott. 1993.
  Includes bibliographical references and index.
  ISBN 0-89079-936-9 (alk. paper)
  1. Drooling. 2. Drooling—Prevention. 3. Saliva. I. Scott, Amanda. II. Johnson, Hilary.
Practical approach to saliva control. III. Title.
  [DNLM: 1. Sialorrhea—prevention & control. 2. Saliva. 3. Salivation—physiology. WI
230 S425p 2004]
RC815.5.J64 2004
616.3'16—dc22

2003069018

This book is designed in Janson Text and Melior.

Printed in the United States of America

1 2 3 4 5 6 7 8 9 10   08 07 06 05 04

Contents

Preface

In the early 1990s, we wrote the first edition of this book to share our knowledge with the wider community. We were naive about the interest in the area, and we have been very pleased with the response to our first edition. In the past 10 years, we have broadened our knowledge in the area but are still a long way from finding the solutions that we seek. The evidence base for this area is still seriously lacking: The general lack of interest from the medical community in seeking to further research in this area has been disappointing. It has been our experience that research submissions that focus on the area of saliva control are rarely successful. Treatments other than medical or surgical need serious research funding if we are to provide evidence based on randomized control groups or good single-study designs. Many people with saliva control difficulties do not have discrete problems but have broad and encompassing disabilities (e.g., cerebral palsy, Parkinson's disease, intellectual disability). The area of saliva overflow is still not taught in most undergraduate or postgraduate courses, and there is little awareness of this difficulty in the research community.

In the early 1990s, a group of pioneers in the United States hosted a seminar to look at the area of drooling. A lateral approach was taken that involved NASA, and the question was asked, "If we can control body fluids on the moon, how come we can't control them on the earth?" This consortium included speech–language pathologists, engineers, medical practitioners, and scientists. Their 2-day meeting resulted in a number of recommendations. Some of these recommendations have been followed through, and we are pleased to include the outcomes from two international instigators of the consortium in this edition of our book. Research moves slowly, and we hope the outcomes of the consortium will be available soon to a wider audience.

Royalties from this book have been placed into a fund for further research. The monies from the sale of the first book have been spent bringing international speakers to Australia. We have seen Professor Hubert Haberfellner, a leading expert, and his partner, physical therapist Ursula Haberfellner, from Austria conduct lectures and seminars. Professor Haberfellner also has helped us set up the Innubruck Sensori Motor Activator and Regulator (ISMAR) project. We also had Professor Colin Dawes, an eminent dentist from Canada, spend several days sharing with us detailed information about saliva. Smaller in-house seminars also have been held with a range of local speakers. For many years we commenced an organization called ANZSCOFD (Australian and New Zealand Society of Oro Facial Disabilities) through which we organized seminars and published several newsletters. This organization was the hard work of just a few people, and so it had a short life span.

Our clients and patients urge us to become better informed. One of the areas in which knowledge has been increasing is information about saliva and what to do when one has too little saliva or there are changes in saliva consistency. This is usually more of an issue for people with progressive disabilities and people on multiple medications, especially those who are aging. This important area has become a much greater part of our work and has resulted in our changing the title of the book to reflect this.

One of the more positive changes for us in Melbourne has been the willingness of dentists to become part of our team. While on a Churchill fellowship just 10 years ago, Hilary attended a conference in Venice on dentistry for children with disabilities. Here began the forging of important links with dentists from Melbourne. The oral-health area is much better represented in this edition, and this representation reflects the broadening of our understanding of team approach and practices.

The embarrassment and social isolation that accompanies drooling often has meant that children and adults avoid certain activities and situations or endure negative community attitudes. For people who, for a number of reasons, are unable to swallow their saliva effectively and regularly, treatment has ranged from developing oral–muscular control to surgically excising the saliva glands or ducts. These treatments often have been applied from a least intrusive to most invasive hierarchy; that is, from assisting with the development of oral sensory–motor control, to behavioral programs and intraoral appliances, and finally to more invasive medical or surgical intervention. This range of intervention has involved speech–language pathologists, occupational therapists, physical therapists, psychologists, dentists, doctors, and surgeons, depending on the courses of action prescribed.

In this book, we present a team approach based on theoretical and clinical expertise. Each chapter commences with learning outcomes to assist the reader. In Chapter 1, we briefly introduce the anatomy and physiology of saliva production and swallowing. In Chapter 2, we outline the impairments that cause difficulties in drooling and saliva consistency. These problems are illustrated by vignettes from people we have met in our clinical practice. (Names have been changed to preserve anonymity.) In Chapter 3, we describe the team members and a number of assessment procedures for children and adults with a saliva loss problem or poor oral hygiene. This chapter was expanded to include not only clinical tools but also other valid and reliable tools that can be used. We also include possible methods of measuring drooling. Chapter 4 is a new chapter, in which we outline the importance of oral health and suggest techniques that might be successful to improve oral health. In Chapter 5, we examine the background of oral–facial facilitation and suggest some oral–motor programs to try. In Chapter 6, we update our approaches to the behavioral management of saliva loss. Chapter 7 is another exciting new chapter written by U.S. authors that introduces new technologies that could assist our research and interventions. Chapter 8 was expanded, and we focus on intraoral appliances. We were fortunate to have Professor Haberfellner help with that chapter and also increase our experience using plates and ISMARs. In Chapter 9, we provide an update of medical management, including the use of radiation and botulinum toxin. In Chapter 10, we outline the surgical approaches for drooling and include previously unpublished results of drooling surgery carried out at the Royal Children's Hospital in Melbourne. In Chapter 11, we expand on the previous edition and include published articles on complementary therapies such as acupuncture.

We did not design this book to be a cookbook of recipes. We offer a framework to assessment and measurement and outline a range of interventions. We provide a list of references for further reading at the end of each chapter. We would like to encourage clinicians and practitioners to consider the importance of publishing single case studies and of examining carefully the efficacy of interventions. We also need to listen closely to people with saliva problems and their caregivers to refine and create better treatments. We hope that people will use our reproducible assessment forms and handouts and respond with suggestions regarding additions that we need to make.

We would like to acknowledge the voluntary work of all authors to produce this new and challenging book. Thanks also to Sue Reid and Katie Hazard, research assistants who worked hard to pull together the surgery data, to Peter King for his case study in Chapter 8, and to Libby Ferguson for reading the first few chapters. We appreciate the contributions of Gloria Staios, Libby Ferguson, Denise West, and Chris Bennett to the first edition of this work. We also are thankful for the loving support we have received from our friends and colleagues, especially Don Scott and Sue Jackson.

Contributors

Janet Allaire, MA
University of Virginia
Kluge Children's Rehabilitation Center
2270 Ivy Road
Charlottesville, VA 22902
United States
E-mail: JHA6E@hscmail.mcc.virginia.edu

Carrie Brown, PhD
Innovative Human Services, Inc.
4636 Cherokee Trail
Dallas, TX 75209-1907
United States
E-mail: cbr949@airmail.net

Margaret Foulsum, BAppSci
Bethlehem Health Care
476 Kooyong Road
South Caulfield 3162
Australia
E-mail: MargF@bethlehem.org.au

Hubert Haberfellner, MD
Children's University Hospital
Anichstrasse.35
A 6020 Innsbruck
Austria
E-mail: Hubert.Haberfellner@uklibk.ac.at

Hilary Johnson, DipSpThy, MA (ed), (FSPAA)
Communication Resource Centre
830 Whitehorse Road
Box Hill 3128
Australia
E-mail: hjohnson.crc@scopevic.org.au

Bruce Johnstone, MB, BS, FRACS
Royal Children's Hospital, 7th Floor
766 Elizabeth Street
Melbourne 3000
Australia
E-mail: bjkr@bigpond.com

Bronwen Jones, BAppSci
SCOPE
44 Alamein Avenue
Ashwood 3147
Australia
E-mail: bronwenjones@ozemail.com.au

Nicky Kilpatrick, BDS, PhD, FDS, RCPS
Department of Dentistry
Royal Children's Hospital
Flemington Road
Parkville 3082
Australia
E-mail: kilpatrick@cryptic.rch.unimelb
.edu.au

James Lucas, BSc, MDSc, LDS, FRACDS, FICD
Department of Dentistry
Royal Children's Hospital
Flemington Road
Parkville 3082
Australia
E-mail: drjameslucas@bigpond.com

Susan Mathers, MB, MRCP, FRACP
Bethlehem Health Care
476 Kooyong Road
South Caulfield 3162
Australia
E-mail: smathers@bethlehem.org.au

Dinah Reddihough, MD, BSc, FRACP, FAFRM
Child Development and Rehabilitation
Royal Children's Hospital
Flemington Road
Parkville 3082
Australia
E-mail: reddihod@cryptic.rch.unimelb
.edu.au

Amanda Scott, BAppSci, PhD
   The Alfred
   Commercial Road
   Prahran
   Australia
   E-mail: A.Scott@alfred.org.au

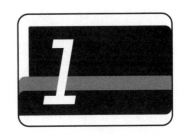

Saliva Production and Swallowing

Learning Outcomes

- *Understand the functions of saliva*
- *Outline the anatomy and physiology of saliva*
- *Describe the flow and distribution of saliva*
- *Appreciate the normal development of teeth*
- *Outline normal swallowing in children and adults*
- *Describe the differences between swallowing saliva and swallowing for nutrition*

To understand the mechanisms that cause drooling and difficulties with saliva, we need a sound knowledge of the role and production of saliva. In this chapter, we outline the importance of saliva, the anatomy and neurology of saliva production, and the development of the oral occlusion and swallowing.

FUNCTIONS OF SALIVA

Saliva has seven major functions:

1. It lubricates food to assist with chewing and turns the food into a bolus for ease of swallowing.

2. It lubricates the tongue and lips during speech.

3. It cleanses the teeth and gums and assists with oral hygiene.

4. It regulates acidity in the esophagus.

5. It destroys microorganisms and clears toxic substances.

6. It facilitates taste.

7. It initiates carbohydrate digestion.

Saliva is important for the health of the mucous membranes of the mouth and pharynx and for gum and oral health. Oral health can be defined as the standard of health of the oral and related tissues that enable an individual to eat, speak, and socialize without active disease, discomfort, and embarrassment and that contribute to general well-being. In terms of the teeth and gingival tissues, a healthy mouth is one that is free from active decay (caries) and in which there is an absence of inflammation. In total, we produce approximately 600 mls of saliva a day (Watanabe & Dawes, 1988b), which we swallow. The secretion and reabsorption of this fluid is vital for maintenance of adequate hydration and is particularly important for the normal functioning of the gastrointestinal tract. Throughout the day and night, the mucous membranes are coated by saliva; more viscous saliva is produced by the sublingual, the submandibular, and the minor salivary glands. This coating provides a protective barrier and keeps the membranes supple. The inability to swallow effectively the saliva produced in the mouth or to produce sufficient amounts of saliva has ramifications for the healthy functioning of the whole body. The reduction of saliva to swallow can lead to dehydration, constipation, and digestive complications.

ANATOMY AND PHYSIOLOGY OF SALIVA

The major salivary glands are the parotid, submandibular, and sublingual glands (see Figure 1.1). The submandibular glands secrete 60% of the total saliva at rest, and the parotid glands secrete 25%. The sublingual and minor mucous glands provide the remaining saliva. The parotid glands secrete saliva through Stenson's ducts near the upper second maxillary molar teeth, the submandibular glands secrete saliva through Wharton's ducts on either side of the frenulum of the tongue, and the sublingual glands secrete saliva through several ducts in the floor of the mouth. There are also many minor glands

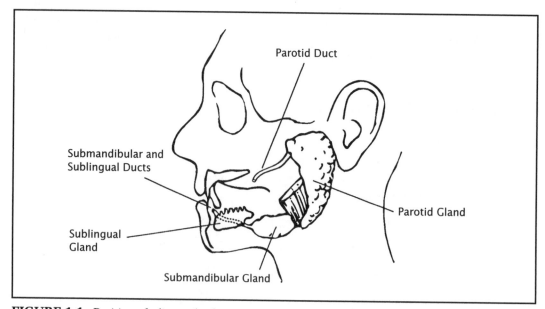

FIGURE 1.1. Position of salivary glands.

found in the mucosa or submucosa of the tongue, palate, and oral cavity. The saliva from minor glands is secreted through very short ducts, unlike the major glands that secrete saliva through ducts away from the gland.

Each pair of major glands produces different types of saliva. The parotid glands produce serous secretions (thin and watery) and are particularly active during eating and drinking. The submandibular glands have serous and mucous secretory cells and produce mainly thin, serous secretions but also some more viscous, mucous secretions. The sublingual glands also are mixed but produce predominantly mucous secretions. Generally, people produce more saliva when they are awake, and there is strong evidence to support definite circadian rhythms. In fact, saliva production peaks in the midafternoon (Dawes & Ong, 1973). It also is possible that we have circannual rhythms, but this has yet to be researched fully (Shannon, 1966).

Saliva coats the inside of the mouth (which has an average surface area of 200 sq. cm) in a very thin film (0.1 mm). It moves backward slightly in the mouth from buccal to lingual surfaces but does not cross over to the other side of the mouth. The speed at which saliva moves is from 0.83 to 7.6 mm per minute. It moves slowest from the buccal to upper incisors and fastest from the lingual to lower incisors. The slower the film of saliva the more likely it is for caries to develop. The velocity is lowest on the buccal aspect of the teeth, thus the buccal surface should be more susceptible to caries than the lingual surface. The surface film velocity is more important in protecting the teeth than is the sugar concentration of saliva in the case of causing smooth surface caries (Dawes, 1997).

There is a wide range of saliva production that is considered normal. Individuals have their own unique patterns of saliva production.

NEUROPHYSIOLOGICAL ASPECTS OF SALIVA PRODUCTION

The complexity of the regulation of saliva production still is not fully understood. The salivary glands are regulated by the autonomic nervous system, which governs involuntary reactions. The influence of the autonomic system means that many factors may influence the salivary flow, such as emotional state and physical pain. External influences, such as eating food, also affect the flow of saliva. The cerebral cortex integrates the effects on saliva flow, which come from internal and external stimuli. There also appears to be an internal homeostatic mechanism that regulates saliva flow. Thus, if for some reason saliva flow is reduced (perhaps by surgical removal of a gland) there may be an increase in the flow of saliva to reinstate the homeostatic balance. The innervation of the saliva glands is summarized in Figure 1.2.

FACTORS INFLUENCING SALIVA PRODUCTION

Other factors that affect the production of saliva are gender, age, hydration, mastication, taste, smoking, sight of food, visualization, mood or psychosis, light, posture, disease and nerve damage, and medication. Examples of these effects are described in the following text.

Gender

The effect of gender is not yet fully explained. Differing results are reported, and the main difference is reported between adults and children, with men producing the most saliva.

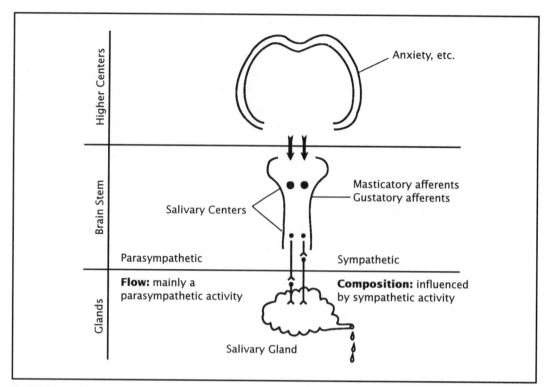

FIGURE 1.2. Neural control of salivary activity. Diagrammatic representation of afferent and efferent pathways that are involved in reflex salivary secretion under the coordinating control of salivary centers. These are in turn influenced by higher centers and, in this manner, anxiety, and so on, may have effects on the reflex flow of saliva.

In some studies of adults (Ghezzi, Lange, & Ship, 2000; Lagerluf & Dawes, 1984), gender differences across whole-mouth saliva have been reported as statistically nonsignificant. However, there is often a trend that indicates men secrete more saliva. Researchers report differences when unstimulated saliva is statistically significant (Bergdahl, 2000; Rudney & Larson, 1995), with a higher volume of saliva reported in men.

Regarding children, reseachers described a gender difference (Andersson, Arviddson, Crossner, Holm, & Mansson, 1974; Crossner, 1984), with girls having lower stimulated flow rates than boys. However, Watanabe, Ohnish, Imai, Kawano, and Igarashi (1995) studied unstimulated whole saliva in 60 five-year-old Japanese children and reported no significant gender-related difference.

Age

Andersson et al. (1974) found that with children, the mean rate of unstimulated and stimulated whole salivary flow increased up to age 15 years. Unstimulated saliva in boys in the 13-year-old age group showed a significantly higher flow rate than did girls in a similar age group. The reason for the increase in saliva flow could again be linked to gland size. As the children increased in age, their gland size also increased and more saliva was produced. Watanabe et al. (1995) estimated total saliva volume to be 500 ml per day in 5-year-old children.

Generally in adults there is little difference in the volume of saliva production before the age of 60 years. Researchers speculate that hormones contribute to rhythmic variations in saliva flow rates (Dawes & Chebib, 1972; Palmai & Blackwell, 1965). This is particularly important in women at or above the age at which they begin menstruation. It may be that the effect of menstruation affects the rate of saliva flow. Puskulian (1972) studied the stimulated flow in a small study that showed a lower flow rate at ovulation than during other parts of the menstrual cycle. Streckfus et al. (1998) stated that the flow rate of stimulated whole saliva was the same for pre- or postmenopausal groups, but unstimulated and stimulated submandibular saliva was greater in the premenopausal group. Ghezzi, Wagner-Lange, et al. (2000) suggested that age may lessen the flow of stimulated parotid saliva. However, a number of menopausal women complain of oral discomfort, which may be due more to the changing constituents of saliva than to its flow (Ben Aryeh et al., 1996).

There is some controversy among researchers on saliva production in the aged population. Frequently it is stated that saliva production decreases. However, when the effects of aged dentition, medication, and disease are controlled, there appears to be a very similar flow rate to that of younger people, especially in stimulated saliva. The effects of losing teeth in older people does pose a problem for eating (Hildebrandt, Dominguez, Schork, & Loesche, 1997), and masticatory function significantly declines with age (Idowu, Grase, & Handleman, 1986). Yeh et al. (2000) confirmed an age-related decrease in the force of the bite and salivary flow rates.

Hydration

The assumption that thirst comes from having a dry mouth is true for some people but not for all. Although recent research is scarce in this area, Holmes (1964) determined that reducing body water content did reduce the unstimulated saliva flow and correlated dehydration with a lessened saliva flow in proportion to the degree of water lost. However, stimulated saliva after mechanical and gustatory influence did not show any influence of the dehydration. Hyperhydration causes an increase in salivary flow rate (Shannon, 1966, 1972; Shannon, Feller, & Suddick, 1972). Because the range of "normal" saliva flow rate is currently broad, general agreement of what is "dry" is important. If a person had a relatively high normal flow rate, a reduction in flow might cause the mouth to feel dry even though saliva flow remained within normal limits. Also, the viscosity of the saliva may be an important factor in the feeling of dryness. Absence of a coating of mucoid saliva can lead to a feeling of dryness in the mouth even when saliva flow is within normal limits (Sreebny & Broich, 1987).

Mastication

There is general acceptance that chewing and biting increases saliva flow (Hector, 1985; Navazesh & Christensen, 1982; Yeh et al., 2000). Hector (1985) recorded the saliva flow of 8 participants who crushed Grape Nuts in their mouths. This cereal was chosen because it is dry, hard, and brittle and considered tasteless. Anesthesia was applied to the periodontal ligament during trials, and a reduction in the saliva flow from the parotid glands was noted during anesthesia. This experiment demonstrated the contribution of the periodontal receptors to saliva flow. Jensen Kjeilen, Brodin, Aars, and Berg (1987) showed salivation increased with frequency and force of chewing. The frequency and force of chewing stimulated the periodontal mechano-receptors, which reinforced their major role in the parotid gland's response to chewing. When there is poor periodontal stimulation (perhaps due to ill-fitting dentures or soft food) a lesser amount of saliva might be produced. These conditions are most frequently found in the elderly population, in institutionalized settings, or among students with oral–motor disabilities (Yeh et al., 2000).

Taste

The study by Jensen Kjeilen et al. (1987) also compared chewing with the influence of taste. Their results showed that salivation increased with frequency and force of chewing but that citric acid produced greater dose-dependent salivary increases than did chewing. Watanabe and Dawes (1988) also compared tasting and chewing on the flow rate of whole saliva with three foods: rhubarb pie, boiled rice, and raw carrot. The effects of taste-elicited salivary flow rates ranged from 73% to 87% of those elicited by chewing.

Combined Influences of Taste and Chewing

Muniz, Maresca, Tumilasci, and Perec (1983) studied the response of parotid saliva to a change in diet among 66 healthy boys who lived in a children's home. The authors' main emphasis was to look at salivary component changes for developing a nutritious and caries-reducing diet. The diet was based on foods (animal protein and fresh fruit and vegetables) that had a 25% overall higher caloric value than the boys' previous diet. There was a 40% reduction in carbohydrates and an increase in fat. After 45 days on the diet, the response of the parotid glands to stimulation was significantly increased by 40% when compared with pretest measures.

Smoking

In general, researchers agree that smoking increases the flow of saliva (Macgreggor, 1988; Pangborn & Sharon, 1971). The overall flow rate could be doubled to that before smoking or upon quiting smoking. Bergdahl (2000) stated that male smokers have a statistically significant lower unstimulated salivary flow than male nonsmokers.

Sight of Food

The sight of food is commonly thought to produce saliva, hence the saying "mouth watering." However, this is not fully borne out in the research. A few studies (Birnbaum, Steiner, Karmell, & Islar, 1974; Christensen & Navazesh, 1984; Wooley & Wooley, 1974) looked at the effects on anticipatory saliva flow in the presence of certain foods. The results varied from no significant difference to one difference related only to certain foods (e.g., pizza and lemon slices).

Visualization

Researchers studied the use of imagery to increase or decrease salivary flow rates (Shannon & Chauncey, 1969; White, 1978; Wooley & Wooley, 1974). On the basis of the results from the study of the parotid gland's saliva, Shannon and Chauncey (1969) suggested that visualization had no effect on salivation, whereas the studies on whole-mouth saliva demonstrated an effect. It appeared that vivid imaging abilities might assist in controlling the saliva flow. This technique to reduce saliva flow is not likely to be useful for people with an intellectual or cognitive disability.

Mood or Psychosis

The knowledge of the effect of emotion on saliva was used long ago in the Indian Rice Test. In this test, a suspect who was unable to swallow his rice because of a lack of saliva was assumed to be afraid of detection and was therefore deemed guilty (Burgen & Emmelin, 1961). Since then, a considerable amount of interest has been shown in the study of the flow rate of saliva in relation to both depressive illness and emotional state. Numerous researchers (Anttila, Knuuttila, & Sakki 1998; Bolwig & Rafaelson, 1972; Busfield, Weschler, & Barnum, 1961; Palmai & Blackwell, 1965) studied the area of psychotic state. Their findings were similar in that a clinically depressive state reduced the saliva flow. Once the person had recovered, the flow returned to normal.

Bergdahl and Bergdahl (2000) studied people who complained of having a dry mouth and found this was significantly associated with "depression, trait anxiety, perceived stress, state anxiety, female gender and the intake of hypertensives" (p. 1652). Stress and anxiety also have been proven to reduce parotid saliva flow. Bogdonoff, Bogdonoff, and Wolfe (1961) compared personality types with the effect of a stressful activity (the approach of the dentist drill). The results of this study suggested that those people rated as more aggressive were more likely to increase their saliva flow in an anxiety-provoking situation, whereas those people whose patterns were more defensive were more likely to exhibit decreased saliva flow.

Light

Shannon, Feller, and Suddick (1971) stated that light influences the flow of parotid saliva, which reinforced the findings of other researchers' work (Barylko-Pikielna, Pangborn, & Shannon, 1986; Pangborn & Sharon, 1971). The flow rate of saliva decreased markedly when blindfolds were used. It might be that light provides the principal stimulus for this basal and continuous rate of resting secretion by the human parotid gland. It might also partly explain why saliva flow reduces during sleep. A study of the effects of blindfolding and blindness (Dong & Dawes, 1995) suggested there were statistical differences in whole saliva reduction between blindfolded, sighted people and controls but not between blind individuals and controls.

Posture

Shannon et al. (1971, 1972) reported that the overall position of participants during standing, sitting, and lying down affected salivary flow rates. Those participants who were standing had the highest flow rates, while those participants lying down had lower flow rates than seated participants.

Disease and Nerve Damage

Diseases that affect the salivary glands have been shown to have an effect on saliva flow. Examples of these diseases include Sjögren's disease, Bell's palsy, tumors on the salivary nucleii, or damage to the vagus nerve or chorda tympani. A reduced flow of saliva often results in a disordered swallow (Fox, Ven, Sonies, Weiffenbach, & Baum, 1985; Hughes et al., 1987).

It also has been suggested that gum disease will increase the amount of saliva in the mouth by increasing the amount of fluid due to irritation of the mucous membranes of the mouth. Gum disease is common among people with oral–motor disabilities (Desai, 1997; Nunn, Gordon, & Carmichael, 1993; Stiefel, Truelove, Persson, Chin, & Mandel, 1993).

Medication

There are more than 400 drugs listed that produce a dry mouth (Sreebny & Schwartz, 1986). Examples include anorectic drugs, anticholinergics, antidepressants, antipsychotics, diuretics, sedatives and hypnotics, antihistamines, antiparkinsonians, and antihypertensives. Many older people receive medications that may cause a dry mouth as a side effect. Thomson, Chalmers, Spencer, and Slade (2000) reported briefly on the use of cholinergic (increase salivation) and anticholinergic (decrease salivation) drugs. Subcutaneous cholinergic stimulation on 6 participants elicited a sixfold increase in saliva from the unstimulated saliva rate. The application of an intravenous anticholinergic on the same 6 participants almost abolished salivation. Some of the medications used to control epilepsy might also increase salivation (Curran, Jardine, & Sharples, 1999; Wyllie, Wyllie, Cruse, Rothner, & Erenberg, 1986).

It is sometimes artificial to separate the factors that affect saliva production, because many of these factors go together; for example, age and gender, medication and disease, and chewing and dentition. Early increase in drooling is often perceived to be due to teething, and certainly irritated gums produce extra saliva. It is important to understand the development of skeletal growth and dentition, because it is related to saliva control during teeth eruption and swallowing when a malocclusion may make lip closure difficult.

THE DEVELOPMENT OF DENTITION

Skeletal Growth

Growth of the jaws (the mandible and maxilla) is related to the growth of the cranium that in turn is related to the growth of the brain. At birth, the cranium is about 65% of its final adult dimensions. About 90% of all the cranium's growth is completed by the age of 5 years. However, the facial skeleton develops much later and is characterized by downward and forward growth during the pubertal growth spurt.

What controls musculoskeletal growth is still unclear, but there is undoubtedly a strong genetic influence. Growth of the craniofacial skeleton is strongly influenced by cartilaginous plates in the synchondroses at the base of the skull. Movement of the plates, along with the activity of the lips, cheeks, tongue, and muscles of mastication, can have a profound effect on the development of the structures of the face. This effect becomes an important factor when considering the potential outcomes of treating the malocclusions in individuals with conditions such as cerebral palsy where there is abnormal muscle activity.

Occlusal Development

Teeth start to form from the 5th week in utero and may continue until the late teens or early 20s with the eruption of the third permanent molars (or wisdom teeth; see Table 1.1). The first teeth to erupt are usually the lower central primary incisors at around 7 months of age. By the age of 2½ years, most children will have complete primary dentition (see Figure 1.3). There is considerable variation in occlusal development, and provided that the sequence of eruption is relatively normal, delayed eruption is not usually of concern.

TABLE 1.1
Eruption Sequence of Primary Dentition (Months After Birth)

Central Incisors		Lateral Incisors		Canines		First Molars		Second Molars	
Lower	**Upper**	**Lower**	**Upper**	**Lower**	**Upper**	**Lower**	**Upper**	**Lower**	**Upper**
6–10	8–12	10–16	9–13	17–23	16–22	14–18	13–19	23–31	25–33

Note. From *Oral Structural Biology*, by H. E. Schroeder, 1991, Stuttgart, Germany: Georg Thieme Verlag. Copyright 1991 by Georg Thieme Verlag. Reprinted with permission.

FIGURE 1.3. Anterior view of complete primary dentition.

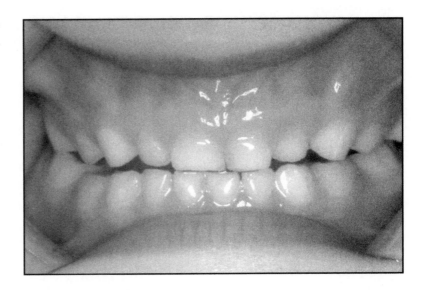

Permanent dentition begins to develop at around the age of 6 years, usually with the eruption of the lower first permanent molar teeth (see Table 1.2). This is followed closely by the upper first permanent molars, the lower incisors, and then the upper incisors. The permanent upper incisors are more proclined than their predecessors, and this allows the mandible to grow forward and encourages the development of a Class I occlusion. The period that follows, referred to as the *mixed dentition phase*, is highly variable, with the eruption of the teeth in the buccal segments beginning around the age of 11 years and culminating in the unpredictable eruption of the wisdom teeth sometime after 18 years of age.

Normal Variation

Figure 1.4a is an example of permanent dentition in a Class I occlusion. Although often described as "normal," this ideal situation is relatively uncommon, and the development of the permanent dentition is frequently neither well organized nor ideal.

Variations of the norm are commonplace, and variation in one structure is often accompanied by a compensatory change in another. Anteroposterior discrepancies are very common and will influence the relative position of the upper and lower anterior teeth or incisors. In cases where the maxilla is forward relative to the mandible, the upper incisors

TABLE 1.2
Eruption Sequence of Permanent Dentition (Years of Age Decimal)

Central Incisors		Lateral Incisors		Canines		First Premolars		Second Premolars	
Lower	Upper	Lower	Upper	Lower	Upper	Lower	Upper	Lower	Upper
6.0–6.9	6.7–8.1	6.8–8.1	7.0–8.8	9.2–11.4	10.0–12.2	9.6–11.5	9.6–10.9	10.1–12.1	10.2–11.4

First Molars		Second Molars		Third Molars	
Lower	Upper	Lower	Upper	Lower	Upper
5.9–6.9	6.1–6.7	11.2–12.2	11.9–12.8	17.0–19.0	7.0–19.0

Note. The decimal point represents a decimal rather than a month. From *Oral Structural Biology*, by H. E. Schroeder, 1991, Stuttgart, Germany: Georg Thieme Verlag. Copyright 1991 by Georg Thieme Verlag. Reprinted with permission.

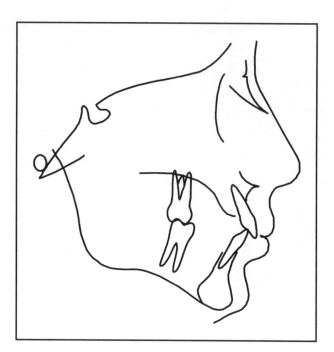

FIGURE 1.4a. An example of permanent dentition in Class I occlusion. *Note.* Courtesy of Chris D. Stevens.

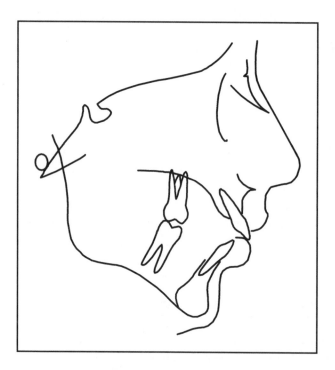

FIGURE 1.4b. Class II skeletal pattern. *Note.* Courtesy of Chris D. Stevens.

appear too far forward in a Class II relationship (see Figure 1.4b). Conversely, in those cases where the mandible is relatively prognathic, the upper front teeth develop behind the lower ones in a Class III relationship (see Figure 1.4c). These malocclusions may result from growth anomalies in either or both jaws and may be further complicated by the pattern of eruption of the dentition, the size of the teeth, and external influences such as thumb sucking.

FIGURE 1.4c. Class III skeletal pattern.
Note. Courtesy of Chris D. Stevens.

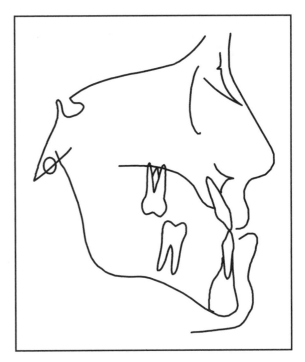

Teething

Teething is an inevitable phase of growth that starts as early as 4 months and continues until the last primary molar teeth have erupted sometime before the age of 3 years. The myths surrounding teething have their roots firmly planted in history, with teething being blamed for any number of childhood diseases since Hippocrates's time. There is no doubt that teething can be uncomfortable for a child, as the gums become reddened and slightly swollen just prior to eruption (Hulland, Lucas, Wake, & Heskeeth, 2000). However, it would appear that many of the symptoms commonly attributed to teething are in fact based on parental perception rather than on clinical experience (Wake, Hesketh, & Allen, 1999). Children certainly do chew objects or their fingers and may drool excessively; however, a direct association with the teething process is unclear (Seward, 1972; Tasanen, 1968). When there is drooling in a young child, teething is often seen as the cause even without evidence of a direct association between teething and drooling. It is rare (with the exception of the commonly impacted third permanent molars) for the eruption of the permanent dentition to be associated with any increased saliva production. Management of issues associated with teething is generally confined to symptomatic approaches such as analgesics and soft diets.

NORMAL SWALLOWING IN THE CHILD

Swallowing is an unconscious act by which we transport saliva, food, or drink from the mouth into the stomach. Swallowing of amniotic fluid commences in utero. When the child is born, the tongue fills the oral cavity and appears large in relation to the oropharynx, as the mandible is small and retracted. The presence of sucking pads in the cheeks help stabilize the jaw. The larynx is high in the neck. Neonates are nose breathers and can swallow and breathe simultaneously. By 4 to 6 months, the sucking pads reduce, the larynx descends, and separate mouth and nose breathing becomes possible. At this time, coordination of breathing and swallowing becomes particularly important, and swallowing difficulties may arise if this coordination is not present. The larynx descends in childhood until it is opposite the sixth cervical vertebra and in adulthood reaches the seventh cervical vertebra. The face grows vertically, and the spaces in the mouth and throat enlarge. This is illustrated in Figure 1.5 (Morris & Dunn-Klein, 2000, p. 52).

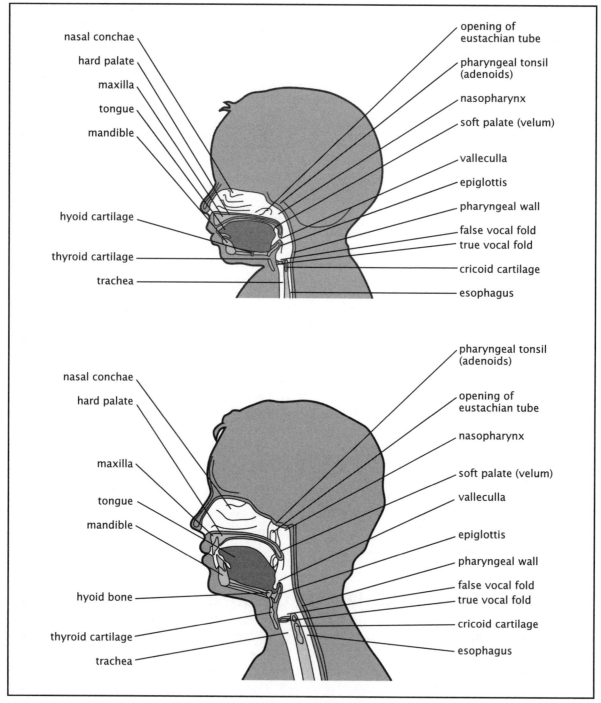

FIGURE 1.5. Anatomical differences between the newborn and the adult mouth and pharynx. *Note.* From *Pre-Feeding Skills: A Comprehensive Resource for Mealtime Development* (2nd ed.), by S. E. Morris and M. Dunn-Klein, 2000, San Antonio, TX: Psychological Corp. Copyright 2000 by Psychological Corp. Reprinted with permission.

TABLE 1.3
Oral Reflexes

Reflex	Stimulus	Age of Onset (Weeks Gestational)	Age of Disappearance (Postnatal Months)
Pharyngeal swallow	Bolus	12	6–12
Suckling	Nipple or stroke top of tongue	18–24	6–12
Gag	Touch	26–27	Persists
Rooting	Touch	28	3–6
Phasic bite	Pressure on gums	40	9–12

Note. Adapted from *Pediatric Swallowing and Feeding*, by J. C. Arvedson and L. Brodsky (Eds.), 1993, London: Whurr.

In the early months after the baby is born, primitive reflexes operate to assist with the infant's survival (see Table 1.3). The rooting reflex orients the baby's mouth to the nipple. During suckling, the lower jaw and tongue move vertically against the palate and upper jaw and also move horizontally, posterior to anterior. Initially, the infant's jaw and tongue operate as single unit, suckling from the breast or the bottle. This action provides negative oral pressure to remove the liquid from the teat or nipple and pumps the liquid down the throat. It is a sucking and a propelling activity. Liquid is sucked over a flattened tongue. Thus, the mouth can be seen as having two parts: the liquid or saliva in the lower part and the upper part where liquid or saliva is sucked up (Lespargot, Langevin, Muller, & Guillemont, 1993).

As the infant grows, so do the oral structures that encourage independent or combined precise movements of the jaw, lips, cheek, and tongue and facilitate the development of a mature swallow. The process of ingestion, chewing, swallowing, and breathing eventually presents as a seamless activity and becomes a mature swallow. Once a child reaches the age of 6 years, the pattern of his or her swallow remains the same throughout young adulthood (Tulley, 1962).

NORMAL SWALLOWING IN THE ADULT

Anticipatory Phase

The anticipatory phase occurs before food or fluid is placed within the mouth. A person's breathing is adapted to ensure that he or she is not inhaling air at the same time as he or she is ingesting food. As food or fluid approaches the lips, a person usually breathes in and then possibly breathes out a small amount of air. This breathing is followed by a period of apnea until the swallow is completed. This period of apnea ensures that the lungs have sufficient air to produce a cough to clear the airway without further inhaling should any of the bolus be aspirated. The structures of the mouth and pharynx assume positions appropriate for ingesting food and fluid. The lips open, the jaw drops, and the tongue rests on the floor of the mouth. The stimulus of food during this period results in an increase in the production of saliva.

Oral Preparatory Phase

The oral preparatory phase of the swallow takes place once the food or fluid is placed within the mouth. The lips close to provide an anterior seal for the bolus. The function of this phase of swallowing varies according to the nature of the bolus. With solid foods, a fragment may be bitten from a larger piece by the anterior teeth. Depending on its texture, the food may then be chewed. Chewing occurs as food is ground by the molars and mixed with saliva as it is moved around the oral cavity by the rotary movements of the jaw and tongue. The soft palate is lowered to touch the back of the tongue to prevent posterior leakage of the bolus into the pharynx. Once the bolus has been modified into a moist, cohesive consistency suitable for swallowing, the bolus is collected onto the dorsum of the tongue. This phase of the swallow is somewhat shorter when the bolus does not require chewing, such as with fluid or purees.

Oral Phase

Once the bolus has been centered on the tongue, the tongue tip elevates and the blade of the tongue then makes contact with the hard palate in an anterior to posterior direction as the bolus is pushed back into the pharynx (see Figures 1.6a and 1.6b). The jaw is stable during this phase and acts as an anchor for tongue movement.

Pharyngeal Phase

The sequential contraction of the pharyngeal constrictor muscles is primarily responsible for the movement of the bolus through the pharynx to the esophagus. During this phase of swallowing, the pharyngeal tube must be closed off from the nasal cavity and from the

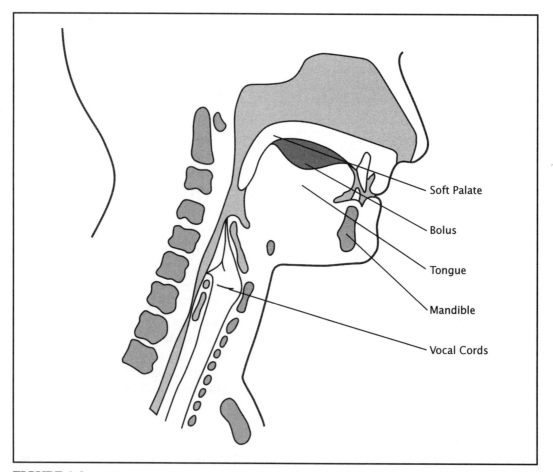

FIGURE 1.6a. Bolus centered on the tongue at the beginning of the oral phase of swallowing.

laryngeal opening to the airway. The soft palate elevates and the superior pharyngeal constrictor contracts to close the nasal cavity from the pharynx, thus maintaining negative pressure within the pharyngeal lumen and preventing nasal regurgitation. Because the pharynx acts as both the upper airway and upper digestive tract, a system of airway protection is activated as the bolus moves through the pharynx. Protection of the airway is achieved by the elevation of the larynx, to reduce the laryngeal opening, the forward tilting of the larynx, and the closure of the vocal folds (see Figure 1.7a). At the lowest part of the pharynx the cricopharyngeal muscle opens to enable the bolus to pass into the esophagus. This sphincterlike muscle is usually in a state of tonic contraction to maintain closure of the esophagus. During the pharyngeal phase of swallowing, this muscle relaxes and is opened by the traction resulting from the elevation of the larynx and cricoid cartilage into which this muscle is inserted (see Figure 1.7b).

Esophageal Phase

This phase of swallowing begins as the bolus passes through the cricopharyngeus to the esophagus. The movement of the bolus through the tube-like structure of the esophagus is brought about by the contraction of the smooth muscle. The lower esophageal sphincter opens to allow the transit of the bolus into the stomach. This normally takes 8 to 20 seconds.

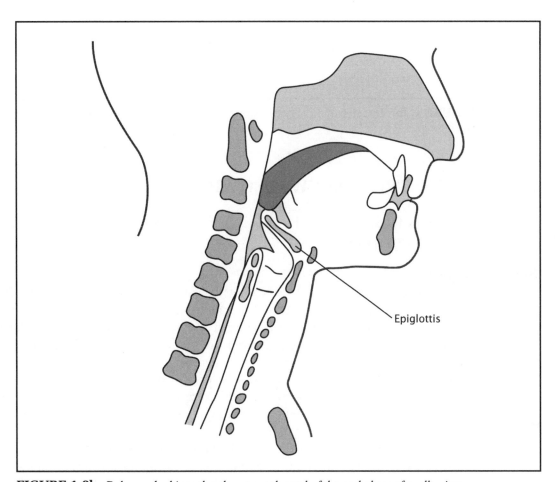

Epiglottis

FIGURE 1.6b. Bolus pushed into the pharynx at the end of the oral phase of swallowing.

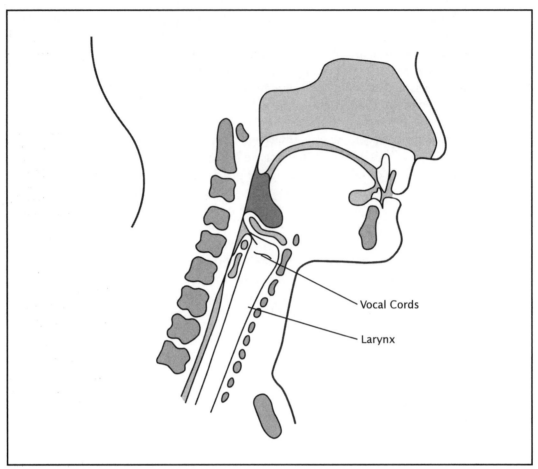

Vocal Cords

Larynx

FIGURE 1.7a. Elevation of the laryngeal structures to protect the airway during the pharyngeal phase of swallowing.

NEURAL CONTROL OF SWALLOWING

The successful execution of the phases of swallowing requires integration of the functions of several cranial nerves.

Sensory Aspects

Adequate oral and pharyngeal sensation is necessary for normal swallowing. In the oral phase of swallowing, the structures of the mouth must detect the presence of material to make the appropriate movements to control and push the material into the pharynx. Information relating to touch and pressure from the lips and oral cavity is conveyed by the sensory division of the trigeminal nerve. This communication provides information relating to the size, shape, and texture of a bolus. Information about the taste of a bolus is mediated by the trigeminal nerve for the anterior two thirds of the tongue and by the glossopharyngeal nerve for the posterior tongue. Information conveyed by the olfactory nerve enhances the perception of taste.

Once the bolus reaches the area of the oropharynx, the involuntary pharyngeal phase of the swallow is initiated. The initiation of the swallow reflex is dependent on adequate pharyngeal sensation to respond to the presence of the bolus in the pharynx. The swallow reflex can be elicited from the faucial region and the laryngeal, pharyngeal, and

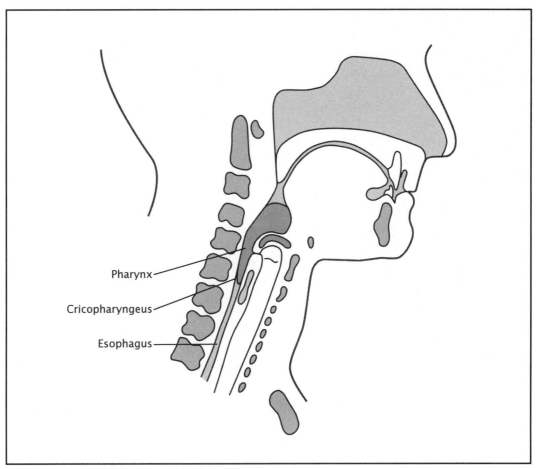

FIGURE 1.7b. Bolus passing through the cricopharyngeus at the end of the pharyngeal phase of swallowing.

epiglottic regions. Pressure receptors of the glossopharyngeal nerve and the superior laryngeal nerve, a branch of the vagus nerve, provide afferent information that triggers the swallow reflex.

Motor Aspects

The facial nerve is responsible for the muscles that maintain the oral seal. Chewing is mediated by the motor division of the trigeminal nerve. During the oral preparatory phase, rotary movements of the tongue move the bolus around the oral cavity. The hypoglossal nerve innervates the tongue muscles. As the bolus is pushed to the back of the oral cavity, the first action of the swallow reflex, the elevation of the soft palate, occurs. This action is primarily mediated by the vagus nerve. Elevation of the hyoid and larynx and forward movement of the larynx are mediated primarily by the trigeminal nerve, with some input from the facial and hypoglossal nerves. The glossopharygeal nerve also contributes to hyoid elevation and also is involved in the dilation of the pharynx with the stylopharyngeus muscle. However, the vagus nerve is the main contributor to the pharyngeal phase of swallowing. Apart from soft palate elevation, the rapid sequence of closure of the laryngeal vestibule by approximation of the vocal folds, ventricular folds, and aryepiglottic folds: contraction of the pharyngeal constrictors; relaxation of the cricopharyngeus; and the initiation of esophageal peristalsis are all functions mediated by the vagus nerve.

SWALLOWING SALIVA

The ability to control saliva flow requires an effective swallow and a frequent swallow. The swallowing processes during a saliva swallow are very similar to that of a food and drink swallow except for the obvious absence of an anticipation phase. What triggers a swallow? The swallowing reflex for food and drink commences at a specific point between the oral and pharyngeal phases, but the triggers are a complex combination of the properties of the bolus, cortical influences, and individual variations (Wolf & Glass, 1992). In addition, the brain stem has a role in swallowing. It is not known if the trigger for a saliva swallow is the same as for a nutritional swallow, but it is possible these are different.

For food and drink, the trigger may lie somewhere from the faucial arches to the vallecula. Nutrition excites our sensory systems by taste, texture, odor, and temperature. Saliva has few of these properties, so the ability to sense very small volumes of liquid, as in saliva, and automatically to swallow relies on an intact sensory system. Here the preparatory phase of the swallow is very important. Murray, Logeman, Larson, and Zecker (2001) studied the interlabial pressure of the labial muscles during swallowing and noted that labial activity was greater for 20 ml swallows than for 1 ml swallows.

Lespargot et al. (1993) suggested that a key factor to assist the swallowing of saliva is the ability to suction liquid to swallow onto the tongue. In their study examining intraoral pressure in swallowing, Lespargot et al. found the normal pattern to be one in which negative suction pressure in the oral cavity is rapidly followed by positive propelling pressure. The swallowing of saliva has not been as rigorously studied as the swallowing of food and drink. This is partly due to the difficulty of imaging the saliva swallow. In most cases, ultrasound has been used to image saliva swallows, but this is not a widely used technique (Sonies, Wang, & Sapper, 1996). More recently, the development of cervical auscultation (Groher, 1995) showed promise for measuring swallowing frequency in different populations (see Chapter 3 for further details).

SWALLOWING RATE

The absence, inadequacy, and infrequency of swallowing is cited in the literature as a major factor (but not the only factor) contributing to saliva loss. There is very little information available on the saliva swallow rates of children. Massengill (1973) found differences on five parameters of swallowing between a small group of young people with intellectual disabilities and a control group. Sochaniwskyj, Koheil, Bablich, Milner, and Kenny (1986) studied three groups of children (12 children in each group): one group with no disabilities, one group with cerebral palsy, and one group who had cerebral palsy and drooled. The authors measured the frequency of swallowing by electromyography, in which electrodes are placed on the muscles involved in swallowing and the resultant activity recorded on a graph. Sochaniwskyj et al. (1986) described that children with cerebral palsy swallowed at 45% of the normal rate. The authors also identified that nondrooling children with cerebral palsy swallowed at 75% of the normal rate. However, Lespargot et al. (1993) found that children with cerebral palsy who drooled swallowed at three times the rate as those who did not drool. Both of these studies had small numbers of participants, thus the results must be interpreted with care. It may be useful to compare the swallowing rate of people with saliva loss to the swallowing rate of people who have adequate saliva control in each specific disability. More important is to understand the disrupted mechanisms that cause drooling in each disability type.

There is a range of swallowing rates recorded for various activities among healthy adults. Even when we consider the area of sleeping, in which the nocturnal swallowing rate seems more uniformly low compared with the daytime swallowing rate (Kapila, Dodds, Helm, & Hogan, 1984; Lear, Flanagan, & Moorrees, 1965; Lichter & Muir, 1975), there are differences. Lear et al. (1965) established there was a wide range of 19 to 90 swallows for different individuals over the same period. Rudney and Larson (1995) reported the range among their dental students to be 0.3 to 6.7 swallows per minute, 4.5 to 100 swallows per 15 minutes, and 18 to 400 swallows per hour. Thus daily estimates are approximate but may mean an individual swallows saliva more than 1,000 times a day. Kapila et al. (1984) administered atropine to healthy adults and noticed their swallow rate reduced significantly after the injections. However, the absence of saliva did not eliminate swallowing, and it was postulated that the participants swallowed in response to the feeling of dryness in their mouths.

Some researchers showed interest in the efficacy and frequency of saliva swallows. We have already pointed out that the saliva flow rate varies from person to person, and Rudney and Larson (1995) stated that, although there are differences in how frequently people swallow, there is a close relationship between individual volume and flow. In Rudney and Larson's study, individuals who combined high flow rates with small saliva volumes had short swallowing intervals. This result suggests that oral clearance might be more efficient for individuals with low flow rates and large saliva volumes, and oral clearance might be related to swallowing frequency. Sonies, Ship, and Baum (1989) suggested that it is not unusual to see healthy persons without major gland unstimulated flow, even though they display swallow times completely in the normal range.

The volume of saliva in the mouth varies between 0.8 ml and 1.1 ml. Salivary flow rate for children is lower than for adults (Watanabe & Dawes, 1990), but the thickness of the film of saliva coating the mouth is similar to that of an adult. When swallowing a residual volume of saliva, between 0.4 and 1.7 ml is left behind in the mouth.

REFERENCES

Andersson, R., Arviddson, E., Crossner, C. G., Holm, A. K., & Mansson, B. (1974). The flow rate and pH buffer effect of mixed saliva on children. *Journal of International Association of Dentistry in Children, 5,* 5–12.

Anttila, S. S., Knuuttila, M. L., & Sakki, T. K. (1998). Depressive symptoms as an underlying factor of the sensation of dry mouth. *Psychosomatic Medicine, 60*(2), 215–218.

Arvedson, J. C., & Brodsky, L. (Eds.). (1993). *Pediatric swallowing and feeding.* London: Whurr.

Barylko-Pikielna, N., Pangborn, R. M., & Shannon, I. L. (1986). Effects of cigarette smoking on parotid secretion. *Archives of Environmental Health, 17,* 731–738.

Ben Aryeh, H., Gottlieb, I., Ish-Shalom, S., David, A., Szargel, H., & Laufer, D. (1996). Oral complaints related to menopause. *Maturitas, 24*(3), 185–189.

Bergdahl, M. (2000). Salivary flow and oral complaints in adult dental patients. *Community Dentistry and Oral Epidemiology, 28*(1), 59–66.

Bergdahl, M., & Bergdahl, J. (2000). Low unstimulated salivary flow and subjective oral dryness: Association with medication, anxiety, depression, and stress. *Journal of Dental Research, 79*(9), 1652–1658.

Birnbaum, D., Steiner, J. E., Karmell, F., & Islar, M. (1974). Visual stimuli and human salivation. *Psychophysiology, 11*(3), 288–293.

Bogdonoff, M. D., Bogdonoff, M., & Wolfe, S. G. (1961). Studies on salivary function in man. *Journal of Psychosomatic Research, 5,* 170–179.

Bolwig, T. G., & Rafaelson, O. J. (1972). Salivation in affective disorders. *Psychological Medicine, 2,* 232–238.

Burgen, T. G., & Emmelin, N. G. (1961). *Physiology of the saliva glands.* London: Edward Arnold.

Busfield, B. L., Weschler, H., & Barnum, W. J. (1961). Studies of salivation in depression. *Archives of General Psychiatry, 5*(11), 472–477.

Christensen, C. M., & Navazesh, M. (1984). Anticipatory saliva flow to the sight of different foods. *Appetite, 5,* 307–315.

Crossner, C. G. (1984). Salivary flow rate in children and adolescents. *Swedish Dental Journal, 8,* 271–276.

Curran, A. L., Jardine, P., & Sharples, P. M. (1999). Gabapentin in paediatric epilepsy: The first 2 years' experience. *Developmental Medicine and Child Neurology, 41*(81), 14.

Dawes, C. (1997, September). *Saliva.* Paper presented at the Australian and New Zealand Care of Orofacial Disabilities, Melbourne, Australia.

Dawes, C., & Chebib, F. S. (1972). The influence of previous stimulation and the day of the week on the concentrations of protein and the main electrolytes in human parotid saliva. *Archives of Oral Biology, 17,* 1289–1301.

Dawes, C., & Ong, B. Y. (1973). Circadian rhythms in the flow rate and proportional composition of parotid to whole saliva volume in man. *Archives of Oral Biology, 18,* 1145–1153.

Desai, M. (1997). *A study of the dental treatment needs of children with disabilities in Melbourne, Australia.* Unpublished master's of dental science thesis, University of Melbourne, Melbourne, Australia.

Dong, C., & Dawes, C. (1995). The effects of blindfolding and blindness on the unstimulated and chewing-gum stimulated flow rates of whole saliva. *Archives of Oral Biology, 40*(8), 771–775.

Fox, P. C., Ven, P. F., Sonies, B. C., Weiffenbach, J. M., & Baum, B. J. (1985). Xerostomia: Evaluation of a symptom with increasing significance. *Journal of American Dental Association, 110,* 509–515.

Ghezzi, E. M., Lange, L. A., & Ship, J. A. (2000). Determination of variation of stimulated salivary flow rates. *Journal of Dental Research, 79*(11), 1874–1878.

Ghezzi, E. M., Wagner-Lange, L. A., Schork, M. A., Metter, E. J., Baum, B. J., Streckfus, C. F., & Ship, J. A. (2000). Longitudinal influence of age, menopause, hormone replacement therapy, and other medications on parotid flow rates in healthy women. *Journals of Gerontology. Series A, Biological Sciences & Medical Sciences, 55*(1), 34–42.

Groher, M. E. (1995, October). *The year in cervical auscultation.* Paper presented at the meeting of the Dysphagia Research Society, McLean, VA.

Hector, M. P. (1985). The masticatory-salivary reflex. In S. J. W. Lisney & B. Matthews (Eds.), *Current topics in oral biology* (pp. 311–320). Bristol, England: University of Bristol Press.

Hildebrandt, G. H., Dominguez, B. L., Schork, M. A., & Loesche, W. J. (1997). Functional units, chewing, swallowing and food avoidance in the elderly. *Journal of Prosthetic Dentistry, 77,* 588–595.

Holmes, J. H. (1964). Changes in salivary flow produced by changes in fluid and electrolyte balance. In L. M. Sreebny & J. Meyer (Eds.), *Salivary glands and their secretions* (pp. 177–195). New York: Macmillan.

Houston, W. J. B. (1982). *Orthodontic diagnosis.* London: Wright P.S.G.

Hughes, C. V., Baum, B. J., Fox, P. C., Marmary, Y., Yeh, C. K., & Sonies, B. C. (1987). Oral-pharyngeal dysphagia: A common sequela of salivary gland dysfunction. *Dysphagia, 1,* 173–177.

Hulland, S. A., Lucas, J. O., Wake, M. A., & Heskeeth, K. D. (2000). Eruption of the primary dentition in human infants: A prospective study. *Pediatric Dentistry, 22,* 415–421.

Idowu, A., Grase, G., & Handleman, S. (1986, March/April). The effect of age and dentition status on masticatory function in older adults. *Special Care in Dentistry,* 80–83.

Jensen Kjeilen, J. C., Brodin, P., Aars, H., & Berg, T. (1987). Parotid salivary flow in response to mechanical and gustatory stimulation in man. *Journal of Physiology Scandinavia, 131,* 169–175.

Kapila, Y. V., Dodds, W. J., Helm, J. F., & Hogan, W. J. (1984). Relationship between swallow rate and salivary flow. *Digestive Diseases and Sciences, 29*(6), 528–533.

Lagerluf, F., & Dawes, C. (1984). The volume of saliva in the mouth before and after swallowing. *Journal of Dental Research, 63*(5), 618–621.

Lear, C. S., Flanagan, J. B., & Moorrees, C. F. A. (1965). The frequency of deglution in man. *Archives of Oral Biology, 10,* 83–99.

Lespargot, A., Langevin, M., Muller, S., & Guillemont, S. (1993). Swallowing disturbances associated with drooling in cerebral-palsied children. *Developmental Medicine and Child Neurology, 35,* 298–304.

Lichter, I., & Muir, R. C. (1975). The pattern of swallowing during sleep. *Electroencephalograph Clinical Physiology, 38*, 427–432.

Macgreggor, I. D. M. (1988). Smoking, saliva and salivation. *Journal of Dentistry, 16*, 14–17.

Massengill, R. M. (1973). Comparison of the swallowing patterns of mental retardates and normals. *American Journal of Mental Deficiency, 78*, 950–955.

Morris, S. E., & Dunn-Klein, M. (2000). *Pre-feeding skills: A comprehensive resource for mealtime development* (2nd ed.). San Antonio, TX: Psychological Corp.

Muniz, B. R., Maresca, B. M., Tumilasci, O. R., & Perec, C. J. (1983). Effects of an experimental diet on parotid saliva and dental plaque pH in institutionalized children. *Archives of Oral Biology, 28*(7), 575–581.

Murray, K. A., Logeman, J., Larson, C. R., & Zecker, S. G. (2001). Interlabial pressure and electromyography in the labial muscles during the oral swallow. *Dysphagia, 16*(2), 148.

Navazesh, M., & Christensen, C. M. (1982). A comparison of whole mouth resting and stimulated salivary measurement procedures. *Journal of Dental Research, 61*(10), 1158–1162.

Nunn, J. H., Gordon, P. H., & Carmichael, C. L. (1993). Dental disease and current treatment needs in a group of physically handicapped children. *Community Dental Health, 10*, 389–396.

Palmai, G., & Blackwell, B. (1965). The diurnal pattern of saliva flow in normal and depressed patients. *British Journal of Psychiatry, 111*, 334–338.

Pangborn, R. M., & Sharon, I. M. (1971). Visual deprivation and parotid response to cigarette smoking. *Physiology Behaviour, 6*, 559–561.

Puskulian, L. (1972). Salivary electrolyte changes during the normal menstrual cycle. *Journal of Dental Research, 51*(5), 1212–1216.

Rudney, J. D., & Larson, C. J. (1995). The prediction of saliva swallowing frequency in humans from estimates of salivary flow rate and the volume of saliva swallowed. *Archives of Oral Biology, 40*(6), 507–512.

Schroeder, H. E. (1991). *Oral structural biology.* Stuttgart, Germany: Georg Thieme Verlag.

Seward, M. H. (1972, Spring). Teething disturbances and their treatment. *Dental Health,* 5–8.

Shannon, I. L. (1966). Climatological effects on human parotid gland function. *Archives of Oral Biology, 11*, 451–453.

Shannon, I. L. (1972). *The biochemistry of human saliva in health and disease.* Paper presented at the Proceedings of a Symposium on Salivary Glands and Their Secretions, Ann Arbor, MI.

Shannon, I. L., & Chauncey, H. H. (1969, July/October). Verbal suggestion and parotid flow. *Journal of Oral Medicine,* 104–108.

Shannon, I. L., Feller, R. P., & Suddick, R. P. (1971). Light deprivation and parotid flow in the human. *Journal of Dental Research, 51*(6), 1642–1645.

Shannon, I. L., Feller, R. P., & Suddick, R. P. (1972). Effects of body position, blood pressure and sleep on human parotid gland function. *Annals of Dentistry, 31*(4), 81–86.

Sochaniwskyj, A. D., Koheil, R. M., Bablich, K., Milner, K., & Kenny, D. J. (1986). Oral–motor functioning, frequency of swallowing and drooling in normal children and in children with cerebral palsy. *Archives of Physical Medicine and Rehabilitation, 67*, 866–874.

Sonies, B. C., Ship, J. A., & Baum, B. J. (1989). Relationship between saliva production and oropharyngeal swallow in healthy, different-aged adults. *Dysphagia, 4*, 85–89.

Sonies, B. C., Wang, C., & Sapper, D. (1996). Assessment of hyoid movement during swallowing by the use of ultrasound duplex-doppler imaging. *Dysphagia, 11*(2), 162.

Sreebny, L. M., & Broich, G. (1987). Xerostomia (dry mouth). In L. M. Sreebny (Ed.), *The salivary system.* Boca Raton, FL: CRC Press.

Sreebny, L. M. & Schwartz, S. (1986). Reference guide to drugs and dry mouth. *Gerodontology, 5,* 75.

Stiefel, D. J., Truelove, E. L., Persson, R. S., Chin, M. M., & Mandel, I. S. (1993). A comparison of oral health in spinal cord injuries and other group. *Special Care in Dentistry, 13,* 229–235.

Streckfus, C. F., Baur, U., Brown, L. J., Bacal, C., Metter, J., & Nick, T. (1998). Effects of estrogen status and aging on salivary flow rates in healthy Caucasian women. *Gerontology, 44*(1), 32–39.

Tasanen, A. (1968). General and local effects of the eruption of deciduous teeth. *Annales Paediatriae Fenniae, 14*(Suppl.), 1–40.

Thomson, W. M., Chalmers, J. M., Spencer, A. J., & Slade, G. D. (2000). Medication and dry mouth: Findings from a cohort study of older people. *Journal of Public Health Dentistry, 60*(1), 12–20.

Tulley, W. J. (1962). Long-term orthodontic results. *Dental Practitioner and Dental Record, 12,* 253–262.

Wake, M. A., Hesketh, K., & Allen, M. A. (1999). Parental beliefs about teething: A survey of Australian parents. *Journal of Paediatric and Child Health, 35*, 446–449.

Watanabe, S., & Dawes, C. (1988a). A comparison of the effects of tasting and chewing foods on the flow rate of whole saliva in man. *Archives of Oral Biology, 33*(10), 761–764.

Watanabe, S., & Dawes, C. (1988b). The effects of different foods and concentrations of citric acid on the flow rate of whole saliva in man. *Archives of Oral Biology, 33*(1), 1–5.

Watanabe, S., & Dawes, C. (1990). Salivary flow rates and salivary film thickness in five-year-old children. *Journal of Dental Research, 69*(5), 1150–1153.

Watanabe, S., Kawano, E., Saito, E., Ueda, M., Nishihira, M., & Igarashi, S. (1990). The study on salivary clearance in children. The volume of saliva in the mouth before and after swallowing. *Japanese Journal of Pedodontics, 28*(2), 391–396.

Watanabe, S., Ohnish, I. M., Imai, K., Kawano, E., & Igarashi, S. (1995). Estimation of the total saliva volume produced per day in five-year-old children. *Archives of Oral Biology, 40*(8), 781–782.

White, K. D. (1978). Salivation: The significance of imagery in its voluntary control. *Psychophysiology, 15*, 196–203.

Wolf, L., & Glass, R. (1992). *Feeding and swallowing disorders in infancy. Assessment and management.* San Antonio, TX: Psychological Corp.

Wooley, S. C., & Wooley, O. W. (1974). Salivation to the sight and thought of food. *Psychosomatic Medicine, 35*(2), 136–142.

Wyllie, E., Wyllie, R., Cruse, R. P., Rothner, A. D., & Erenberg, G. (1986). The mechanism of nitrazepam-induced drooling and aspiration. *New England Journal of Medicine, 314*(1), 35–38.

Yeh, C. K., Johnson, D. A., Dodds, M. W., Sakai, S., Rugh, J. D., & Hatch, J. P. (2000). Association of salivary flow rates with maximal bite force. *Journal of Dental Research, 79*(8), 1560–1565.

Impairments in Saliva Control and Saliva Consistency

Learning Outcomes

- *Understand how impaired oral function results in drooling*
- *Recognize the effect of pharyngeal dysfunction on saliva control*
- *Describe xerostomia and its impact on the oral cavity*
- *List the reasons for dental caries and gum disease*

There is a range of problems associated with impaired saliva production and control. Individuals experience poor saliva control for many reasons, some of which have been the subject of rigorous investigation. Sensory and motor impairment affecting the oral control of saliva results in drooling. Pharyngeal impairment leads to retention of saliva and pharyngeal secretions and the risk of aspiration. In this chapter, we describe the factors involved and discuss their relationship to drooling in people with acquired and developmental disabilities. Combinations of these factors occur in developmental and acquired populations, however, and the cluster of features may be different. We provide examples of problems associated with specific populations. We also discuss problems associated with an excessively dry mouth (xerostomia) and the presence of thick, tenacious secretions. We also include a discussion on the effect of reduced saliva production and poor oral control on oral health.

THE PROBLEM OF DROOLING

Researchers do not think drooling is due to the overproduction of saliva; rather, they consider it primarily a problem of oral function. Much of our understanding of the factors involved in saliva control comes from work with people with physical or intellectual disabilities, or both, for whom drooling can be an ongoing and lifelong problem. *Drooling, dribbling, saliva overflow,* and *poor saliva control* are all words that conjure up a fairly negative picture. People think of it as a temporary stage in infancy that will disappear as the child grows up, usually resolving between the age of 18 months and 5 years (Blasco,

1996; Brodsky, 1993). Morris and Dunn-Klein (2000, p. 85) stated that babies produce very little saliva until they are 3 months old, but by the age of 2 years they develop the sensory motor skills to control their saliva even when engaged in other motor activities. Some babies are seen as "dribbly" babies, whereas other children take much longer to master saliva control. Recently, Johnson, King, and Reddihough (2001) reported a study wherein some typical children continued to drool until 8 years old. Developmental screening tests (Bayley, 1969; Brigance, 1985; Frankenburg & Dodds, 1975) do not document any developmental stages in saliva control in typically developing children nor the age at which the mastery of saliva control is obtained. It is generally agreed that in infancy, dribbling is not seen to be a problem, but as children enter preschool, problems with saliva control may label children as different, causing embarrassment for them and their peers.

Drooling in adults also can occur. This can occur when people have a developmental disability, oral surgery, brain injury, or a progressive illness in which the ability to control the saliva may be caused by a neurological deficit. In addition, adults with neurological trouble may have trouble managing their secretions. Saliva may become viscous and sticky. Prevalence rates for drooling in children with cerebral palsy vary from 10% (Ekedahl, 1974) to 37% (Van De Heyning, Marquet, & Creten, 1980). In a recent study of people with complex communication needs, 29% presented with saliva control difficulties (Perry, Reilly, Bloomberg, & Johnson, 2002). There are no separate prevalence rates available for those with an intellectual disability or with other neurological conditions.

The range of oral problems that contribute to drooling can encompass poor oral sensation and perception (Drabmen, Corduay y Cruz, Ross, & Lynd, 1979; Weiss-Lambrou, Tétreault, & Dudley, 1989), inadequate oral suction (Lespargot, Langevin, Muller, & Guillemont, 1993), incomplete lip closure (Ray, Bundy, & Nelson, 1983), and infrequent swallowing (Sochaniwskyj, Koheil, Bablich, Milner, & Kenny, 1986). Other factors are frequently associated with the problem of drooling. These factors include lung disease, poor oral health (Scannapieco, 1999), and head-down posture (Thomas-Stonell & Greenberg, 1988).

ORAL DYSFUNCTION AND DROOLING

Saliva is produced within the mouth and swallowed automatically every few minutes throughout the day (Lear, Flanagan, & Moorrees, 1965). As a consequence, impairment of the oral phase of swallowing dysfunction is frequently associated with drooling. Oral function can be impaired in a variety of ways. There may be a problem with an individual's perception, integration, and interpretation of sensory information. An individual's inability to execute the motor program for swallowing (apraxia of swallowing) also can result in drooling. Impairment of the oral phase of swallowing due to weakness or incoordination, or both, of the muscles involved with swallowing almost always co-occurs with speech problems, or dysarthria. This co-occurrence is because the impairment is a neuromuscular problem affecting the structures that serve swallowing and speech. The severity of the salivary control problem is related to the severity of impairment of the swallowing mechanism.

SENSORY PROBLEMS

In some cases, particularly in cerebral palsy, an individual may not have a severe swallowing difficulty but may have a severe drooling problem. The presence of food or fluid on the blade of the tongue seems to provide the extra stimulus needed to execute a swallow successfully, whereas a gradual buildup of saliva under the tongue does not stimulate a swallow. When this is combined with a tongue thrust pattern it can result in a marked drooling problem. When laryngeal and pharyngeal sensation is reduced, the normally protective cough reflex may not be elicited when part of the bolus enters the airway and "silent" aspiration of the bolus occurs.

It has been estimated that 50% to 72% of children with cerebral palsy have sensory disturbances (Menier, Forget, & Lambert, 1996). For some children and adults with a developmental disability, their ability to manage food and drink may be within normal limits, yet they have problems with saliva overflow. They are often seen as messy eaters or people who refuse food that requires sustained chewing (e.g., apple, meat). The primary difficulty for these children may be inadequate sensory feedback. Poor sensory feedback may manifest as hypersensitivity (very sensitive to touch) or hyposensitivity (often unaware of touch). It seems that children with drooling problems may not feel the saliva (hyposensitive) because they often appear not to notice it as it runs down the chin. Consider this in relation to having an injection at a dentist and having part of your face numb. In this situation, there is often no awareness of the saliva and overcompensation by continual dabbing of the handkerchief to ensure there is no dribbling. Weiss-Lambrou et al. (1989) examined oral sensation in a study comparing two groups of children with cerebral palsy: one group with a dribbling problem and one group without. Tests of oral stereognosis (McDonald & Aungst, 1970), oral form discrimination (Ringel, Burk, & Scott, 1970b), and two-point lingual discrimination (Ringel, Burk, & Scott, 1970a) were carried out on the two groups. Lower scores were attributed on all tests to the group of children who drooled; however, only statistically significant results were demonstrated on the oral stereognosis test. The authors caution establishing a causal relationship because of other variables; however, it is likely that impaired sensory perception may be a factor leading to poor saliva control.

Swallowing Apraxia

Although the term *swallowing apraxia* was first used in 1941 by Tuch and Neilson to describe a patient who presented with intact sensation and motor skills but total inability to speak or swallow, the concept of a specific swallowing apraxia is contentious (Daniels, 2000). The problem is described as an inability to perform the usually automatic motor sequence of the oral phase swallowing. People with swallowing apraxia may place food in their mouths but not initiate the oral movements associated with the collection of the bolus onto the tongue and then the backward propulsion of the bolus into the pharynx during swallowing. In some cases, chewing may be initiated but the individual may be unable to progress onto the next aspect of the swallowing sequence, and continue to chew.

 CASE STUDY

Jane, a 35-year-old woman, lost bilateral sensation of the floor of her mouth and tongue following the extraction of her lower wisdom teeth. The lingual nerves, which mediate sensation to those regions, run very close to the lower wisdom teeth and consequently are at risk of damage during wisdom teeth extraction.

Because she is unable to detect the presence of saliva in her mouth until it reaches the areas with sensation, she will sometimes drool. This problem is a source of distress. This is particularly a problem when she is singing, a pastime she previously enjoyed.

She has developed a range of behaviors to compensate for the sensory deficit. In particular, she maintains buccal tension and holds the corners of her mouth tightly closed to reduce the likelihood of drooling. This in turn leads to more generalized muscle tension in her face and neck, which affects the temporomandibular joint and the trapezius and sternocleidomastoid muscles. This tension results in pain and fatigue. She avoids social interaction and is depressed.

This case demonstrates the importance of oral sensation in saliva control. Most people have experienced this problem after a visit to the dentist, but the permanent loss of sensation creates permanent and far-reaching problems.

Apraxia has been defined as an impairment of a learned skilled movement that is not caused by muscle weakness, movement disorders, comprehension deficits, disturbances in sensation, or cognitive disorders (Liepmann, 1997). Other forms of apraxia affecting oral and facial functions—apraxia of speech and buccofacial apraxia, respectively—have been well described in the literature. Apraxia of speech is considered to be a dysfunction of articulation due to difficulty positioning the muscles of speech and sequencing movement (Darley, Aronsen, & Brown, 1975). Buccofacial apraxia is an impairment of the production of oral postures on command or in imitation, with no decrease in involuntary production. Some aspects considered to be characteristic of apraxia of swallowing are also features of apraxia of speech. These aspects include initiation problems and groping lingual movements when an individual is given the command to swallow (Daniels, 2000). Groping lingual movements characteristic of apraxia of speech have been attributed to disturbances in spatial–temporal organization of motor programs (Kent & Rosenbeck, 1983).

It has been argued that some aspects of swallowing apraxia are not typical of apraxias in general. Rothi, Heilman, and Watson (1985) did not consider swallowing a learned skilled movement and therefore should not be considered a form of apraxia. Mature swallowing patterns are not present at birth but develop as the structures subserving swallowing function grow. The extent to which learning contributes to the refinement of movement patterns of swallowing has not yet been established. It is important to note that in speech, as in swallowing, the movement patterns become automatic. However, the principle difference between speech and swallowing is the added complexity of the relationship between thought, language, and speech. The contribution of volition in the execution of the oral phase of swallowing has not been studied extensively.

Gisel, Alphonce, and Ramsay (2000) investigated the relationship between eating and drinking skills and oral praxis skills in children with cerebral palsy. They found that children with cerebral palsy performed tasks of oral praxis, such as the ability to accurately imitate gestures involving jaw, facial, soft palate, and tongue movements, consistently poorer than did children without any neuromotor deficits. Children with cerebral palsy were found to have the most difficulty with tasks that required repetition and smooth sequencing of movements. The authors concluded that impairment of oral praxis contributes a significant component to eating and drinking efficiency.

  CASE STUDY

Jenny is a 15-year-old girl with athetoid cerebral palsy. She uses an electric wheelchair to get around, and her speech is difficult to understand. She also finds eating and drinking a chore and is often embarrassed by her spilling of food and drink. She uses a computer for recording her schoolwork and communicates extensively by e-mail. She can control her drooling in the morning but after lunch it gets more difficult to control. She is trying to arrange her timetable so that she can do more independent study in the afternoon so others do not notice her drooling as much. She is beginning to feel excluded by her friends when they go out on Saturday nights. She has tried to use some medication to control her drooling but hates the dryness of her mouth and finds she wants to drink more. She has had a lot of therapy over the years and finds speech pathology no longer useful. The demands of the day are heavy and she gets tired. As the day wears on she finds it difficult to control her saliva. Most of all, her dribbling embarrasses her. She is looking for a quick and easy solution.

Inadequate Lip Closure

An individual's inability to maintain a good lip seal results in drooling. In some cases this problem may be present often. Other people experience this problem only when they are concentrating on another activity, especially when they are required to have their head and neck in flexion, such as when reading or drawing. Poor lip closure may be caused by flaccid weakness, when the lips are floppy and soft and are unable to maintain a strong seal, or spastic weakness, when the muscles are tight and retracted. Typically the lips of an individual with spastic lip weakness cannot be brought together. Impaired lip closure may coexist with a dental malocclusion, particularly an anterior open bite in which the anterior teeth never form a patent seal. Individuals with a history of persistent colds and the presence of large tonsils and adenoids sometimes develop a habit of holding their tongue forward in their mouth to maintain an unobstructed airway.

 CASE STUDY

Mary is a 53-year-old woman with amyotrophic lateral sclerosis. She presents with spastic retracted lips and a weak atrophied tongue with fasciculations. As a result of these impairments, she is unable to maintain adequate lip closure and cannot use her tongue to collect and push the saliva into her pharynx to be swallowed. Secretions pool under her tongue, and when she leans forward, drooling becomes a problem.

The problem is most apparent when she leans forward to use the keyboard of her communication device, thus requiring a plastic keyboard guard.

Tongue Function

Tongue function is the primary component of the oral phase of swallowing. Tongue impairment can be a result of different types of problems.

Tongue Weakness

The tongue is involved in the collection of saliva within the mouth and the transport of saliva from the mouth into the pharynx. This function can be impaired in a number of ways. The tongue may be flaccid, immobile, and wasted, as frequently occurs in people with ALS, or the tongue may be spastic with reduced strength and range of movement, typical of individuals with pseudo bulbar palsy. In both cases, the outcome of tongue impairment is that saliva within the mouth is not collected onto the tongue and pushed back into the pharynx. This in turn results in a buildup of saliva in the mouth and subsequent drooling.

Tongue Size

It is not uncommon for macroglossia (or large tongue) to be cited as the cause of drooling. However, this view is too simplistic. Occasionally an individual will present with true macroglossia (e.g., Beckwith-Wiedermann Syndrome), however most cases of macroglossia are in fact only "relative macroglossia." In the case of relative macroglossia with muscle hypotonia, the tongue appears to be too large for the mouth (Hoyer & Limbrock, 1990). It is important to understand this concept when considering management of drooling, because interventions such as simply correcting the malocclusion or surgically reducing the tongue are unlikely to have a successful outcome.

Tongue Thrust

Individuals with developmental disabilities often fail to develop a mature pattern of tongue movement during swallowing. During the oral phase of a mature swallow, the bolus is collected onto the blade of the tongue. This is followed by elevation of the tongue tip behind the top front teeth. Finally, the blade of the tongue contacts the roof of the mouth in an anterior to posterior direction to push the bolus into the pharynx. When food is placed in the mouth during a tongue thrust swallowing pattern, the individual pushes the tongue surface toward the roof of the mouth, the teeth, and the lips using a pumping movement instead of using the usual pattern of bolus collection. This movement can result in food or saliva being pushed out of the mouth during the oral phase of swallowing rather than backward to the pharynx and the esophagus. A strong, persistent tongue thrust often results in the front teeth being pushed forward, causing an anterior open bite to develop. This anterior open bite can contribute to poor lip closure.

A milder tongue thrust swallow is often seen in individuals with low muscle tone and intellectual disabilities. Although the tongue may not protrude from the mouth during swallowing, the mild tongue thrust pattern still results in saliva being pushed forward in the mouth.

Fucile et al. (1998) observed increased tongue thrust in the elderly when they drank from a cup. It was not clear why this pattern of tongue movement was exhibited because it was seen more often in the 60-year-old age group than in those individuals who were 80 or 90 years old. The authors considered it was either a habitual behavior (previously undiagnosed) or a compensatory behavior, because oral sensation was diminished.

Impaired Jaw Function

Problems with jaw occlusion can have implications for the management of oropharyngeal secretions. The jaw is a principal point attachment for the muscles of the face, oral cavity, and neck. Functions such as lip closure, tongue tip elevation, and laryngeal elevation rely on jaw stability for optimal movement. These functions are necessary for efficient swallowing and saliva control.

Problems of oral control of saliva may be secondary to jaw or dental malocclusion, or both. The persistent pressure of the thrusting tongue can lead to orthodontic problems, in particular an anterior open bite which results in an inability to occlude the teeth. This in turn can result in an inability to attain or maintain adequate lip closure (see Figure 2.1). Similarly children with a severe overbite may have problems bringing their lips together, which may make keeping saliva inside the mouth difficult (see Figures 2.2a and 2.2b).

FIGURE 2.1. Photo of anterior open bite.

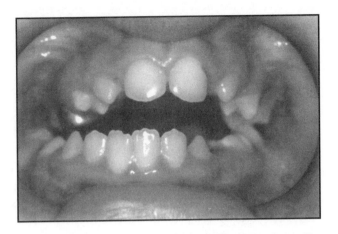

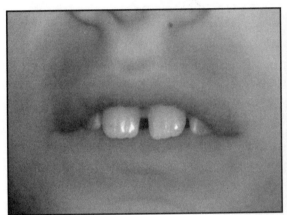
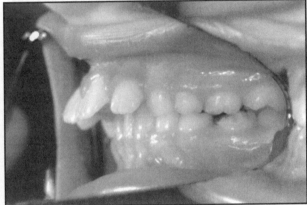

FIGURES 2.2a & 2.2b. Front and side views of an overbite.

The prevalence of malocclusion is high among children with intellectual or physical disabilities, or both (Oreland, Heijbel, & Jagell, 1987; Oreland, Heijbel, Jagell, & Persson, 1989). However, it is important to bear in mind that many individuals have gross skeletal discrepancies but have no problems controlling their saliva. Rather, individuals who drool nearly always have symptoms of oromotor dysfunction in addition to the malocclusion. There is little or no evidence that malocclusion alone causes drooling.

A persistent tongue thrust also can be related to instability of the jaw. These individuals have difficulty initiating the elevation of the pharyngeal structures during the pharyngeal phase of the swallow, because these structures are dependent on jaw stability to provide an anchor point. Swallowing can be effortful and inefficient.

Alignment of the jaw assists an individual's ability to chew. Pelegano, Nowysz, and Goepferd (1994) hypothesized that as individuals with cerebral palsy aged their eating and drinking skills deteriorated, and this was due to contractures of the temporomandibular joint. Thirty-seven participants with spastic quadriplegia and a control group were compared in this study. It was demonstrated that individuals with cerebral palsy had contractures of the temporomandibular joint with overbite being one of the most prominent features. Those participants with an anterior open bite were also more likely to have a gastrostomy for feeding and to have the most severe oral disabilities.

CASE STUDY

John is 9 years old and attends a special class in a mainstream school. He is a cheerful boy with a ready smile and he loves attention. He cannot speak but uses some key word signs to communicate. He never sits still for long. He has an open mouth posture and a tongue thrust swallow, and he is developing a marked anterior open bite. He drools constantly. His teachers find it difficult to deal with, as his work is always wet. The other children also find his drooling on their work or their clothes offensive. His parents have taken him to a dentist to see if there is a plate he can use to help close his mouth. The dentist said there is nothing they can do as his anterior open bite is caused by his tongue thrust. The dentist was reluctant to fit a plate because of John's intellectual disability and his short attention span.

PHARYNGEAL FUNCTIONS AND SALIVA CONTROL

Once saliva has reached the pharyngeal region, the next phase of swallowing begins. During the pharyngeal phase, food or saliva is transported through the pharynx and cricopharyngeal sphincter and into the esophagus. The first element of the involuntary phase is the elevation of the soft palate and constriction of the nasopharynx. As this happens, the laryngeal structures elevate to reduce the size of the laryngeal opening, the epiglottis tilts downward to cover the laryngeal opening, and the glottis closes. These aspects of the pharyngeal phase of swallowing protect the airway from aspirated material. Constriction of the pharyngeal wall provides the propulsive force to transport the bolus through the pharynx.

Impaired Soft-Palate Function

The soft palate plays an important role in the maintenance of negative pressure generated within the oropharyngeal lumen during the transport of food or saliva from the mouth to the pharynx. The elevation of the soft palate in combination with upper pharyngeal constriction closes the oropharyngeal space from the nasal cavity. This closure stops air from escaping through the nose during swallowing, preventing dissipation of negative pressure generated during the transport of the bolus. Failure to close the oropharyngeal space from the nasal cavity also can lead to nasal regurgitation of the bolus during swallowing.

Impaired Pharyngeal Function

Contraction of the constrictor muscles of the pharynx pushes the bolus through the pharynx into the esophagus. When these muscles are weak or uncoordinated, material such as saliva is retained in the pharynx. Because pharyngeal clearing cannot be visualized, pooling of secretions may be present even when swallowing is evident. A wet, gurgly sounding voice can indicate that the airstream associated with speech production is passing through retained secretions. An individual with a persistent wet voice should have his or her swallowing function assessed and his or her chest status closely monitored because there is a risk that retained pharyngeal secretions may be aspirated.

Impaired Cricopharyngeal Function

Retention of secretions in the pharynx can occur because the cricopharyngeus muscle does not open or because the cricopharyngeal opening is not coordinated with the propulsion of the bolus by the pharyngeal muscles. This problem can occur in isolation, particularly after a brainstem stroke. In this case, the individual needs to constantly spit out their secretions that would otherwise pool in the lower pharynx and increase the risk of aspiration.

Impaired Airway Protection

The pharynx is a common pathway for ingested food and fluid, which enters the esophagus, and air, which enters the lungs. It is important that food and fluid not enter the lungs, as that could lead to chest infections. Airway protection is achieved by a series of actions that comprise the pharyngeal, or reflexive, phase of swallowing. When the swallow reflex is initiated, the larynx rises and tilts forward and the vocal folds adduct. These actions reduce the size of the opening to the airway. The opening to the airway is further protected by the epiglottis, which is lowered over the airway. Adequate range and coordination of movement are required to achieve airway protection.

Impairment of the pharyngeal phase of swallowing may lead to aspiration of saliva, which can result in lung infections. Although many people aspirate some saliva, daily exercise and the ability to cough effectively usually dislodges the saliva, and infections do not set in. For people who are frail, have a weak cough, or have very little physical movement, saliva in the lungs can be potentially dangerous. Langmore et al. (1998) and Scannapieco (1999) pointed out the dangers of developing respiratory infections secondary to aspiration of saliva, particularly when oral care is poor and saliva contains pathogens (Terpenning et al., 2001). Potential for aspiration of saliva always has been a concern for surgeons when reducing saliva loss by redirecting saliva ducts into the pharyngeal area. Poor swallowing ability may allow the saliva into the lungs. Stevenson, Allaire, and Blasco (1994) reported on the deterioration and final death of a young woman after surgery for saliva control. Prior to the surgery for saliva control she appeared healthy. After the operation she developed pneumonia and eventually died.

 CASE STUDY

Giovanni, a 42-year-old man with a developmental intellectual disability, is experiencing repeated episodes of pneumonia. He has a history of severe epilepsy, but it has been controlled in the past few years. Recently he moved to a group home because his parents were no longer able to care for him. The videofluoroscopy indicated delayed swallow reflex, particularly with thin fluids. He is slow to initiate a swallow but can manage food with a coarser texture. After speaking to the staff at his house, it appears that they thin down his food to speed up his eating. His mother reported that he likes spicy food, and once the staff at the house experimented with providing him tastier, textured food he began to eat much quicker. His episodes of pneumonia seem to be connected with times after a seizure. Staff were given training to help identify his seizures, and they completed a support manual to indicate Giovanni's food preferences and safe textures.

GASTROESOPHAGEAL REFLUX DISEASE

Gastroesophageal reflux disease (GERD) is a common complaint in Western society for between 5% and 20% of the population. Among children and adults with oral motor difficulties, GERD is even more common in individuals with neurological disabilities (Böhmer, 1996). The incidence in people with neurological impairment may be as high as 75% (Tuchman, 1988).

GERD results when acid from the stomach refluxes into the esophagus and pharynx. This reflux is due to an inadequate lower esophageal sphincter function. Some medications, such as anticonvulsants, can affect the sphincter. Disabilities such as spastic quadriplegia or scoliosis may negatively influence the muscle tone of the sphincter. Repeated incidents of reflux can result in damage to the esophagus, and ulceration and bleeding may develop. Refluxed stomach acid may also enter the pharynx, larynx, and mouth and cause irritation of the mucosa of these structures and consequently increase secretions. In some cases, it may cause vomiting. Erosion to the teeth caused by acid reflux into the mouth leads to an increase in the amount of saliva and bacteria in the mouth. If the individual is dysphagic, this mix of acid and bacteria can be aspirated and is particularly damaging to the lungs.

Heine, Catto-Smith, and Reddihough (1996) hypothesized that GERD may exacerbate drooling by stimulation of the esophagosalivary reflex. However, they found that there was no statistical significant difference in the drooling in participants with both drooling and reflux once GERD was controlled by medication.

 CASE STUDY

Lee Kwan is a 34-year-old woman who has lived in a large institution all her life. Her medical file states she has a profound intellectual disability of no known origin. She has no formal means of communication and has a specially molded wheelchair because of her scoliosis. Her eating began to deteriorate 2 years ago. She started to lose weight and she developed pneumonia. The hospital suggested a gastrostomy and further investigations revealed GERD. This resulted in a fundoplication, a surgical procedure that tightens the lower esophageal sphincter. Her head is forward on her chest and she drools continually. The caregivers have put a plastic-lined protector under and over her clothes. She develops a large stain on her clothes, which have to be changed regularly. There is a marked increase in saliva production after gastrostomy feeding.

XEROSTOMIA AND SWALLOWING DYSFUNCTION

Xerostomia, or dry mouth, is frequently encountered following radiation therapy (Logemann et al., 2001) and in conditions such as Sjögren's syndrome (Schoofs, 2001). This condition leads to problems including ropy tenacious secretions, poor oral health, and swallowing problems.

Sjögren's Syndrome

This condition is a chronic autoimmune disorder in which lymphocytes invade the exocrine, or mucous-producing, glands. This invasion leads to inflammation and progressive loss of lubrication. Reduced lubrication has damaging effects on the eyes, mouth, skin, gastrointestinal tract, ears, nose, and vagina. Extraglandular symptoms occur in approximately one third of sufferers with involvement of the joints, lungs, blood vessels, and nervous and lymphatic systems. The diagnosis of this condition is often difficult because symptoms can be vague and the onset insidious. The full picture may not be recognized because various health professionals may be attending to different aspects of the syndrome. Although it can affect all age groups, middle-aged women are the most frequently affected (Schoofs, 2001).

Viscosity and Flow of Saliva

Each of the salivary glands produces different consistencies and amounts of saliva. Thick and ropy saliva is often difficult to swallow and is unsightly when it crusts on the lips. The minor glands produce mucus saliva. The viscosity of the saliva affects the flow of the saliva in the mouth. The viscosity of the saliva can be affected by what is eaten. Dairy products have been shown to increase the viscosity of saliva (Enderby, 1995).

Saliva has an important role in normal swallowing. It coats the mucosa of the mouth and pharynx, which lubricates these structures and facilitates the transport of the bolus. During the oral preparatory phase of swallowing, saliva is secreted through the parotid glands directly into the region of the second molars. Chewing and tongue movements enable the saliva from the parotid glands to moisten the bolus and contribute to the formation of a cohesive bolus that is easy to swallow. Consequently, xerostomia frequently results in poor bolus formation and difficulties with the oral or pharyngeal transport of the bolus (Hughes et al., 1987).

Impaired oral function can result in the xerostomia. Oral dryness, particularly dryness of the tongue, palate, and oropharynx, occurs when the tongue is unable to disperse saliva around the mouth to lubricate the oral structures.

Persistent mouth breathing also contributes to the problem. Xerostomia is usually at its worst during the night or on waking after a prolonged period of mouth breathing combined with the circadian decrease in saliva production.

An individual may also experience the dual problems of oral dryness and drooling. Drooling occurs because the tongue cannot collect the saliva and transport it into the pharynx to be swallowed. The saliva pools under the tongue and overflows. Xerostomia occurs because the tongue is not able to distribute saliva around the mouth.

Case Study

James is a 70-year-old former company director who has had Parkinson's disease for about 10 years. From diagnosis until his retirement 5 years ago, he had responded well to medication and had experienced only minimal disruption to his life. Since retirement, the number of medications he has taken has gradually increased. He and his wife, Marjorie, have adapted along the way with some aspects of daily living slowly getting more difficult. Although both James and Marjorie had their emotional ups and downs, they have maintained contact with old friends and family. However, over the past 6 months, there has been a more dramatic decrease in his response to medication. The benefits of the medication are occuring for shorter and shorter periods of time. Often, during an "off" period when he is not responding to the medication, he just sits without being able to initiate any activity. His posture has become permanently stooped, his limbs are rigid, he has a marked lack of facial movement, and he also experiences difficulty swallowing his meals.

During these "off" periods, he usually sits in a chair in his lounge room. His mouth is always open and head and neck bent down. There is a lack of spontaneous swallowing, and saliva flows unabated onto his clothing and the furniture. He and his wife find this very distressing. When asked about the impact of the problem, he reports, "It's embarrassing that a person like me, who has achieved many great things in his life, could be drooling. It's foreign to me, you know." His wife adds, "It's changed our social lives, you see. Suddenly, he starts to dribble then … woosh!"

To add to the problem, he is experiencing xerostomia as well. He is having periods when he drools while his mouth feels uncomfortably dry. This xerostomia occurs because the saliva, which pooled under his tongue, is simply lost from his mouth because gravity exerts a greater force than his immobile tongue can. His mouth breathing and anticholinergic medications leave him with a dry, uncomfortable tongue and mouth. His secretions are tenacious and thick, which makes them even more difficult to swallow.

Although drooling and dry mouth were particularly difficult to cope with, James views these problems in the context of his disease, saying, "Well, it's a problem and I don't like doing it [drooling], but it's one of the many problems. There are times that I can't even walk or talk, and I'm frozen. That's more serious to me."

DENTAL CARIES

Dental caries is an infectious disease caused by the presence of certain bacteria (mutans streptococci) that metabolize fermentable carbohydrates (and sucrose in particular) to make acid, which in turn dissolves the enamel surface causing pitting (precavitation). The mutans streptococci bacteria accumulate in the absence of adequate tooth brushing to form dental plaque. Plaque was defined as "the soft non-mineralized bacterial deposits which form on teeth that are not adequately cleaned" (Löe, 1969, p. 679). This soft white layer (which comprises 70% microorganisms and 30% food debris) adheres to dental hard tissue and serves to retain the acid produced by the mutans streptococci against the enamel. Within 3 minutes of the consumption of sugar, the pH in plaque drops significantly and demineralization occurs. It takes about 40 minutes for the pH of plaque to return to its original value; however, this will depend on the amount and thickness of the plaque layer and the volume and buffering ability of the saliva present in the mouth. If sucrose is ingested frequently, the pH of the plaque will remain at a level sufficient to cause demineralization for a longer period of time. The initial signs of demineralization are "white spot" lesions. Early identification of these precavitated areas is important, because they signal the need for proactive preventive measures to encourage remineralization. Failure to change the oral environment to one that encourages remineralization will result in cavities. Once this has occurred, restoration (fillings) is inevitable. There is a high degree of individual susceptibility to dental caries. Table 2.1 summarizes the factors associated with caries risk.

 CASE STUDY

Antoinette is a 12-year-old girl with Angelman's syndrome. She has always drooled copiously. Her parents worked with a speech–language pathologist and tried brushing and icing techniques. Behavioral techniques such as getting Antoinette to follow commands and close her lips were unsuccessful. Eventually her parents were referred to an ear, nose, and throat surgeon who relocated her submandibular ducts and also ligated her parotid ducts. Her parents were very pleased with the result. About 18 months later they noticed some brown spots on her teeth and took her to a dentist. Antoinette does not like brushing her teeth or going to the dentist, and it was difficult to look into her mouth. The dentist found caries on the inside of her front canine teeth, a direct result of the duct relocation surgery. With a careful and stringent oral-hygiene program, the parents were able to protect Antoinette's remaining teeth.

GUM DISEASE

Chronic gum disease (gingivitis) is a nonspecific inflammatory lesion of the marginal gingivae (gums) that reflects the bacterial challenge to the host when dental plaque accumulates in the gingival crevice (Heasman & Murray, 2001). Dental plaque starts to accumulate around the teeth immediately after toothbrushing. If brushing does not occur or is ineffective, the gums mount a subclinical inflammatory response within 2 days that will become clinically apparent in 10 days. The characteristic signs of chronic gingivitis include red, inflamed gums that bleed when brushed and that can deteriorate until there is

TABLE 2.1
Caries Risk Factors

Risk Factor	Influence
Sucrose exposure	Although often very difficult to assess, dietary factors are probably the most significant factor in caries development, with frequency and timing of ingestion being the most highly influential.
Fluoride exposure	Regular exposure to low levels of fluoride can significantly increase resistance of teeth to decay. Fluoridated toothpaste and systemic water fluoridation are the two most effective and common sources of topical fluoride.
Oral-hygiene practices	Presence of dental plaque is an indicator of inadequate toothbrushing and reduced exposure to toothpaste (and thus low levels of topical fluoride). Poor oral hygiene also predisposes people to gum disease.
Levels of cariogenic bacteria	Poor oral hygiene predisposes teeth to plaque buildup, which is associated with higher levels of mutans streptococci. Because caries is essentially an infectious disease, there is a significant risk of transmission from parents, particularly in a young child.
Medical conditions	Exposure to sugar-containing medications predisposes teeth to caries. Poor growth often seen in children with complex medical conditions is often addressed by parents and the medical profession by encouraging high-calorie diets that inevitably are high in sugar.
Disability	Presence of a physical or intellectual disability, or both, can compromise oral hygiene practices. Dysphagia is commonly associated with poor oral clearance and soft diets that predispose individuals to keep food in the mouth longer.
Saliva	The amount, flow, and buffering capacity all influence caries risk. Some medical conditions (e.g., postradiotherapy) and some medications (e.g., antipsychotics) are associated with reduced salivary flow.
Social and family practices	Family practices and attitudes strongly influence a child's risk of developing disease. For example, prolonged (after 12 months of age) and at-will bottle- or breast-feeding is strongly associated with increased caries experience.

bleeding while eating and, in some cases, even spontaneous bleeding. Almost everyone experiences some gingivitis, particularly during adolescence when hormonal changes appear to increase susceptibility (Sutcliffe, 1972). However, chronic gingivitis is relatively easily reversed with good oral hygiene practices to remove the dental plaque.

If left untreated, chronic gingivitis may progress to periodontitis in which the relatively simple inflammatory response within the gingival tissues that characterizes gingivitis becomes a more destructive process within the underlying supporting tissues. This process can lead to significant bone loss around the teeth and accounts for up to 30% of all dental extractions. There is a very high degree of individual susceptibility to periodontal disease, with certain subgroups being particularly prone to destructive periodontal disease, for example, individuals with Down syndrome. Oral disease has implications for general health, including an association with peptic ulcers, respiratory and cardiovascular illness, and increased rates of aspiration pneumonia through contamination of saliva (Terpenning et al., 2001).

PATHOLOGIES OF THE SALIVARY GLANDS

There are several conditions that directly affect the salivary glands, the most common symptoms being pain and swelling. It is important to establish which glands are involved. Problems may be limited to one gland; however, there are systemic disorders that may affect several or all the salivary glands. Mumps is the most common cause of bilateral pain and swelling of the parotid glands. Occasionally the submandibular glands also are involved. Enlargement of the major salivary glands is also associated with the human immunodeficiency virus.

Sialadenitis

Infection of the salivary glands (sialadenitis) may be acute or chronic. Acute infection of the parotid gland is common in older, debilitated patients who are dehydrated and have poor oral hygiene. The glands become swollen and tender, and pus may be observed at the parotid duct. The submandibular glands are less often affected. Treatment usually entails a course of high-dose antibiotics, rehydration, and oral hygiene. If left untreated, a parotid abscess may develop, which would require surgical drainage.

Changes to the architecture of the salivary glands can result in chronic sialadenitis. This usually affects the submandibular glands and may begin insidiously or follow an acute infection. Episodes of pain and swelling after meals are common. Prompt treatment of acute infections is necessary. In severe cases, surgical excision is the only management option.

Sialolithiasis

The formation of stones (calculi) within the salivary glands is more commonly found in the submandibular glands. The thicker, more calcium-rich secretions produced in the submandibular glands may account for this. Sialolithiasis often co-occurs with chronic sialadenitis. Characteristically there is postprandial swelling and tenderness. It is sometimes possible to palpate calculi in the floor of mouth. Diagnosis is usually made by using a sialogram. This entails an X ray of the region following an injection of a radio-opaque dye into the ducts of the salivary gland. Treatment is usually conservative, focusing on hydration and stimulation of salivary flow using sialogogues such as lemon drops. If the problem does not resolve, surgical removal of the calculi from the duct or removal of the gland may be necessary.

REFERENCES

Bayley, N. (1969). *Bayley Scales of Infant Development*. New York: Psychological Corp.

Blasco, P. A. (1996). Drooling. In P. B. Sullivan & L. Rosenbloom (Eds.), *Feeding the disabled child* (pp. 92–105). London: Mac Keith.

Böhmer, C. J. M. (1996). *Gastro-oesophageal reflux disease in intellectually disabled individuals*. Amsterdam, the Netherlands: VU University Press.

Brigance, A. H. (1985). *Brigance Preschool Screen for three and four year old children*. North Billerica, MA: Curriculum Associates.

Brodsky, L. (1993). Drooling in children. In J. C. Arvedson & L. Brodsky (Eds.), *Pediatric swallowing and feeding: Assessement and management* (pp. 390–415). London: Whurr.

Daniels, S. K. (2000). Swallowing apraxia: A disorder of the praxis system. *Dysphagia, 15*(3), 159–166.

Darley, F. L., Aronsen, A. E., & Brown, J. R. (1975). *Motor speech disorders*. Philadelphia: W. B. Saunders.

Drabmen, R., Cordua y Cruz, G., Ross, J., Lynd, S. (1979). Suppression of chronic drooling in mentally retarded children and adolescents: Effectiveness of a behavioural treatment package. *Behaviour Therapy, 10*, 46–56.

Ekedahl, C. (1974). Surgical treatment of drooling. *Acta Oto-Laryngologica, 77*, 215–220.

Enderby, P. C. E. (1995). The effect of dairy products on the viscosity of saliva. *Clinical Rehabilitation, 9*(1), 61–64.

Frankenburg, W. K., & Dodds, I. (1975). *Denver Developmental Screening Test: Reference manual*. Denver: University of Colorado Medical Center.

Fucile, S., Wright, P. M., Chan, I., Yee, S., Langlais, M., & Gisel, E. G. (1998). Functional oral motor skills: Do they change with age? *Dysphagia, 13*, 195–201.

Gisel, E., Alphonce, E., & Ramsay, M. (2000). Assessment of ingestive and oral praxis skills: Children with cerebral palsy vs. controls. *Dysphagia, 15*, 236–244.

Heasman, P. A., & Murray, J. J. (2001). Periodontal diseases in children. In R. Welbury (Ed.), *Paediatric dentistry* (2nd ed., pp. 217–240). Oxford, England: Oxford University Press.

Heine, R. G., Catto-Smith, A. G., & Reddihough, D. S. (1996). Effect of antreflux medication on salivary drooling in children with cerebral palsy. *Developmental Medicine and Child Neurology, 38*, 1030–1036.

Hoyer, H., & Limbrock, J. G. (1990). Orofacial regulation therapy in children with Down syndrome, using the methods and appliances of Castillo-Morales. *Journal of Dentistry for Children, 57*, 442–444.

Hughes, C. V., Baum, B. J., Fox, P. C., Marmary, Y., Yeh, C. K., & Sonies, B. C. (1987). Oral-pharyngeal dysphagia: A common sequela of salivary gland dysfunction. *Dysphagia, 1*, 173–177.

Johnson, H., King, J., & Reddihough, D. (2001). Children with sialorrhoea in the absence of neurological abnormalities. *Child: Care, Health and Development, 27*(6), 591–602.

Kent, R. D., & Rosenbeck, J. C. (1983). Acoustic patterns of apraxia of speech. *Journal of Speech and Hearing Research, 26*, 231–249.

Langmore, S. E., Terpenning, M. S., Schork, A., Chen, Y., Murray, J., Lopatin, D., & Loesche, W. (1998). Predictors of aspiration pneumonia: How important is dysphagia? *Dysphagia, 13*(2), 69–81.

Lear, C. S., Flanagan, J. B., & Moorrees, C. F. A. (1965). The frequency of deglution in man. *Archives of Oral Biology, 10*, 83–99.

Lespargot, A., Langevin, M., Muller, S., Guillemont, S. (1993). Swallowing disturbances associated with drooling in cerebral-palsied children. *Developmental Medicine and Child Neurology, 35*, 298–304.

Liepmann, H. (1997). The syndrome of apraxia (motor asymboly) based on a case of unilateral apraxia. In D. Rotenberg & F. H. Hockberg (Eds.), *Neurological classics in modern translations* (pp. 155–181). New York: Hafner.

Löe, H. (1969). Present day status and direction for future research on the aetiology and prevention of periodontal disease. *Journal of Periodontal Research, 40*, 678–682.

Logemann, J. A., Smith, C. H., Pauloski, B. R., Rademaker, A. W., Lazarus, C. L., Colangelo, L. A., et al. (2001). Effects of xerostomia on perception and performance of swallow function. *Head and Neck, 23*(4), 317–321.

McDonald, E. T., & Aungst, L. F. (1970). An abbreviated test of oral stereognosis. In J. F. Bosma (Ed.), *Second symposium on oral sensation & perception* (pp. 384–390). Springfield, IL: Thomas.

Menier, C., Forget, R., & Lambert, J. (1996). Evaluation of two-point discrimination in children: Reliability, effects of passive displacement and voluntary movement. *Developmental Medicine and Child Neurology, 38*, 523–537.

Morris, S. E., & Dunn-Klein, M. (2000). *Pre-feeding skills: A comprehensive resource for mealtime development* (2nd ed.). San Antonio, TX: Psychological Corp.

Oreland, A., Heijbel, J., & Jagell, S. (1987). Malocclusions in physically and/or mentally handicapped children. *Swedish Dental Journal, 11*, 103–119.

Oreland, A., Heijbel, J., Jagell, S., & Persson, M. (1989, January/February). Oral function in the physically handicapped with or without severe mental retardation. *Journal of Dentistry for Children, 1*, 17–25.

Pelegano, J. P., Nowysz, S., & Goepferd, S. (1994). Temperomandibular joint contractures in spastic quadriplegia: Effect on oral skills. *Developmental Medicine and Child Neurology, 36*(6), 487–494.

Perry, A., Reilly, S., Bloomberg, K., & Johnson, H. (2002). *An analysis of needs for people with a disability who have complex communication needs.* Melbourne, Australia: La Trobe University.

Ray, S. A., Bundy, A. C., & Nelson, D. L. (1983). Decreasing drooling through techniques to facilitate mouth closure. *American Journal of Occupational Therapy, 37*(11), 749–753.

Ringel, R. L., Burk, K. W., & Scott, C. M. (1970a). Oral region two-point discrimination in normal & myopathic subjects. In J. F. Bosma (Ed.), *Second symposium on oral sensation & perception* (pp. 309–320). Springfield, IL: Thomas.

Ringel, R. L., Burk, K. W., & Scott, C. M. (1970b). Tactile perception: Form discrimination in the mouth. In J. F. Bosma (Ed.), *Second symposium on oral sensation & perception* (pp. 410–415). Springfield, IL: Thomas.

Rothi, L. J. G., Heilman, K. M., & Watson, R. T. (1985). Pantomime comprehension and ideomotor apraxia. *Journal of Neurology, Neurosurgery and Psychiatry, 48*, 207–210.

Scannapieco, F. A. (1999, July). Role of oral bacteria in respiratory infection. *Journal of Periodontal Research, 70*, 793–802.

Schoofs, N. (2001). Seeing the glass half full: Living with Sjögren's syndrome. *Journal of Professional Nursing, 17*(4), 194–202.

Sochaniwskyj, A. D., Koheil, R. M., Bablich, K., Milner, K., & Kenny, D. J. (1986). Oral motor functioning, frequency of swallowing and drooling in normal children and in children with cerebral palsy. *Archives of Physical Medicine and Rehabilitation, 67*, 866–874.

Stevenson, R. D., Allaire, J. H., & Blasco, P. A. (1994). Deterioration of feeding behaviour following surgical treatment for drooling. *Dysphagia, 9*(1), 22–25.

Sutcliffe, P. (1972). A longitudinal study of gingivitis and puberty. *Journal of Periodontal Research, 7*, 52–58.

Terpenning, M. S., Taylor, G. W., Lopatin, D. E., Kerr, C. K., Dominguez, B. L., & Loesche, W. J. (2001). Aspiration pneumonia: Dental and oral risk factors in an older veteran population. *Journal of the American Geriatrics Society, 49*(5), 557–563.

Thomas-Stonell, N., & Greenberg, J. (1988). Three treatment approaches and clinical factors in the reduction of drooling. *Dysphagia, 3*(2), 73–78.

Tuch, B. E., & Neilson, J. M. (1941). Apraxia of swallowing. *Bulletin Los Angeles Neurological Society, 6*, 52–54.

Tuchman, D. N. (1988). Dysfunctional swallowing in the paediatric patient. *Dysphagia, 2*, 203–208.

Van De Heyning, P. H., Marquet, J. F., & Creten, W. L. (1980). Drooling in children with cerebral palsy. *Acta Oto-Rhino-Laryngologica Belgica, 34*(6), 691–705.

Weiss-Lambrou, R., Tétreault, S., & Dudley, J. (1989). The relationship between oral sensation and drooling in persons with cerebral palsy. *American Journal of Occupational Therapy, 43*(3), 155–161.

CHAPTER 3

Assessment and Measurement Approaches for Saliva and Saliva Control

Learning Outcomes

- *Describe possible team members and the importance of a team approach*

- *Outline nine areas to consider when assessing drooling*

- *List a number of commercially available assessments for research purposes*

- *Use clinical tools for assessing drooling and secretions*

- *List approaches for further understanding assessments for saliva, saliva overflow, and swallowing frequency*

Over the past few years, the development of technologies has assisted researchers with their understanding of swallowing and saliva. There are now clinical tools, valid assessment procedures, and emerging technological approaches that guide the decision-making process. In this chapter, we introduce reproducible forms for saliva control assessment and secretion assessment in a clinical situation. For clinicians who may want more detail or need validated tools, we outline several other tools. The importance of having a team approach to ensure appropriate investigations occur cannot be overemphasized.

TEAM APPROACH

The remediation of drooling can involve many people, and a team approach provides the best management. Teams may vary in composition depending on the disability type. For instance, the Saliva Clinic at Royal Children's Hospital in Melbourne (Reddihough, Johnson, & Ferguson, 1992) serves children with developmental disabilities and other children. This team comprises a pediatrician, plastic surgeon, speech–language pathologist, and dentist who meet together with the client. Other specialists, such as the otolaryngologist, are accessed by referral. We describe the roles of possible team members in this section. Team members are listed in alphabetical order.

Dentist. A dentist traditionally undertakes the professional assessment of oral health and oral-hygiene practices. The dentist's role is to examine teeth, gums, and dentures and undertake necessary procedures to achieve the best possible oral health for that individual, which might include referral to a dental hygienist to teach a person how to keep teeth and gums healthy. A dental technician may be enlisted to make dental prostheses or to provide denture adjustment, reline, and repair. In some circumstances, the dentist may refer patients to specialist practitioners such as a periodontist (gum specialist), prosothodontist (prostheses specialist), or orthodontist (alignment of jaw and teeth).

Doctor. A doctor or general practitioner may be the first point of referral for a drooling problem. This person will probably make a referral to a specialist such as a pediatrician, an otolaryngologist, or a speech–language pathologist.

Occupational Therapist. Occupational therapists may have specialized knowledge in eating and feeding assessment and treatment. They also may provide expertise in sensory–motor facilitation, positioning, and behavioral techniques related to saliva management.

Pediatrician. This is a medical specialist for children. This person may provide treatment but also will make referrals to other appropriate sources.

Physical Therapist. This person will probably be involved with seating modifications when a physical disability is associated with the drooling. The physical therapist also may be involved with biofeedback as a treatment intervention.

Psychologist. Behavioral psychologists are often helpful in devising programs to decrease unwanted behavior. They also may help structure a program to maximize the person's learning ability.

Neurologist. This person has a detailed knowledge of the nervous system and is a specialized physician; the neurologist is particularly involved with the prescription of medication.

Radiologist. This is a doctor who specializes in diagnosis and therapeutic imaging. These procedures may include investigations with technetium scanning and videoflsuroscopy.

Speech–Language Pathologist. A speech–language pathologist is an expert practitioner in the oral–motor area and is involved with assessment and therapeutic management. The speech–language pathologist will be involved with a detailed eating and drinking assessment.

Surgeon. The surgeon experienced in the area of saliva control is likely to be either a plastic surgeon or a head and neck surgeon. Not all surgeons will be experienced in this area. Some surgeons may use laser techniques.

Complementary Medicine

There are many different types of complementary practitioners who may claim to cure drooling. Usually their work is not underpinned by careful research with people with disabilities. Some of these practitioners include hypnotherapists, acupuncturists, shiatsu therapists, chiropractors, and naturopaths. These practitioners may be of some help but will probably not provide a team approach and may have limited medical knowledge.

HOW TO ASSESS DROOLING

There are four assessment forms provided in Appendix A: Saliva Control Assessment, Drooling Rating Scale, Post–Saliva-Surgery Form, and Oral Secretion Assessment are primarily used with people with developmental disabilities. These forms can be used as a guide and should be completed with as much detail as possible. If the client who drools is unable to complete the form, it is best filled in by a person familiar with the client, such as a parent or teacher. The assessments have been devised to aid decision making regarding appropriate methods of treatment. Measurement is considered an integral part of the intervention process. (See case study examples for decision making.)

The area of saliva control currently lacks a valid and reliable measurement tool. The assessments presented in this chapter are being used clinically but are not statistically valid. They provide questions that might lead to further investigations in particular areas. We encourage you to use these assessments, and we appreciate any feedback. We also refer you to commercially available assessments that cannot be reproduced in this book for copyright reasons.

USING THE SALIVA CONTROL ASSESSMENT FORM

Each area of the form is outlined in the following section along with a rationale for including it. This rationale may help you with the decision-making process for treatment.

Communication Skills (Speech)
People with saliva control problems frequently have difficulty speaking due to reduced oral skills. There are many standardized tests of articulation, and any speech–language pathologist will be able to evaluate this skill. Inadequate saliva control is frequently associated with communication difficulties (Perry, Reilly, Bloomberg, & Johnson, 2002).

Mobility
Although mobility has no obvious connection to saliva control, recent research (Gisel, Schwartz, Petryk, Clarke, & Haberfellner, 2000) indicated improvement in walking after improving the stability of the jaw. Thomas-Stonell and Greenberg (1988) stated that good mobility was one of three factors strongly associated with successful treatment for saliva control.

Head Position
A head-down position often results in saliva pouring out of the mouth. If the answers to Item 3 suggest the person who drools has a problem with head control, it might be necessary to involve a physical therapist for advice. He or she can give suggestions that may assist in the development of head control. If the person can hold his or her head up but continually drops the head, some behavior management advice may be useful (see Chapter 6). Environmental modifications also may be necessary (see Chapter 11).

Oral–Motor Abilities
Items 4, 5, and 6 probe the person's ability to competently use his or her mouth and lips. If the mouth is open all the time, it may be that the person breathes through the mouth and

needs to keep it open. It is possible to mouth breathe without drooling (15% of the population do it). However, if this is the main cause of the drooling, see Chapter 5, Chapter 6, and Chapter 8.

In the case of the person who finds it impossible to bring the lips together, see Chapter 6, Chapter 9, and Chapter 10. When the inability to achieve lip closure is due to a malocclusion, the problem needs to be discussed with a dentist or orthodontist. Items 7 and 8 investigate eating and drinking abilities. When there is any difficulty, a full eating assessment should be carried out to investigate if improved eating skills can be developed. See Chapter 5.

Swallowing

Item 9 relates to the swallowing process. Sometimes the person needs to be taught to swallow more frequently or more effectively (see Chapter 6 and Chapter 8). Sometimes the person is not cognitively able to understand the process of swallowing (see Chapter 9 and Chapter 10).

Sensory Feedback

Items 10 and 11 investigate sensory feedback. If the person cannot feel the saliva on the lips, it will be very difficult to control. When sensory loss is around the outside of the mouth, see Chapter 5, Chapter 6, and Chapter 8 for ideas.

General Health

Items 14 and 15 probe the general health status. It may be necessary to perform an eating assessment for specialist and nutritional advice when general health is poor. Drooling can increase when a person is sick, and the improvement of health must commence before drooling treatment starts. Frequent colds, asthma, and allergies may indicate that the person mouth breathes. It may be necessary to refer the person to an ear, nose, and throat specialist or some other type of medical specialist for further assessment (see the Team Approach section at the beginning of this chapter).

Regular medications also may affect the health status. Some medications for epilepsy can increase drooling; the name and dosage of medications should be noted.

Frequency of Drooling

Items 16 and 17 look at when the drooling occurs. The information should reinforce answers to other scale items and should indicate the effects of physical position, fatigue, concentration, illness, medication, emotional state, and self-stimulatory behaviors.

It is important to ascertain whether the drooling is due to the mouthing of objects or is actually drooling. To do this, it is necessary to observe the person when nothing is in his or her mouth. Some people may need to be restrained physically to keep the mouth free of objects. When the drooling is due predominantly to self-engagement, read Chapter 6. Some children are showing improvement when the drooling is intermittent. Intermittent drooling also may indicate some underlying neurological activity that may need further neurological assessment.

Dental Health

Item 18 requires a full dental assessment, which is helpful in determining if poor dental health may be contributing to the drooling (spongy gums often produce more saliva). A dentist can contribute greatly to the maintenance of good dental health. A full assessment will also comment on the state of the dentition and the occlusion (bite). When there is a large space between the front teeth on the upper and lower jaw, it is important to know if orthodontics will be able to correct the malocclusion. People who have a strong tongue thrust swallow may not be considered for braces or other corrective treatment. In the absence of a dentist, see the section on oral health assessment in this chapter.

Overall Importance of the Saliva Problem

Often people with saliva difficulties have other physical or learning difficulties. It is important to ascertain how severe the saliva problem is. Although the saliva is unsightly, it poses no real health risks. For medically compromised individuals, saliva might not be the most important consideration.

The two case studies provide examples of how the Saliva Control Assessment form can be used to solve problems.

 CASE STUDY

Brendan, age 4 years, has a moderate intellectual disability and presents with a saliva control problem. Brendan

- can keep lips together (Item 5)
- is unable to pucker lips for a kiss and gives an open mouth kiss (Item 6)
- is unable to suck through a regular straw (Item 8)
- pushes tongue out when he swallows (Item 7)
- needs food to be mashed (Item 9)
- is usually healthy and is not on medication (Items 14, 17)
- has occasional dry days with no drooling (Item 16)
- has good occlusion according to dental report (Item 19)

Drooling ratings were frequency 3 and severity 4.

Age and eating difficulties indicated that intervention for Brendan's eating problems should be the first place to start. This also may be coupled with oral–motor skills work, including wearing the vestibular screen while sleeping (see Chapter 8).

 CASE STUDY

Kiara, a 15-year-old girl with multiple and severe disabilities, presents with a severe saliva control problem. Her parents reported that Kiara had extensive intervention to improve her eating skills with little success. She has no functional speech or formal communication system. Kiara

- is not mobile

- has always drooled and has no dry days (Item 15)

- is limited in her ability to keep her head up (Item 3)

- has her mouth habitually open (Items 4, 5, 6)

- eats a soft diet due to her inability to chew (Item 9)

- wears scarves to protect her clothes and changes six or seven times a day (Item 12)

- has no history of chest infections (Item 14)

- has a moderate malocclusion that the dentist concluded would not improve, however she has good dental health (Item 15)

- has epilepsy that is currently controlled by medication (Item 17)

Drooling ratings were frequency 4 and severity 5.

Because of her age and inability to control her saliva physically or intellectually, Kiara would not be able to take an active part in intervention. Surgery was suggested and the pros and cons outlined (see Chapter 10). If, however, Kiara had poor oral health (Item 15), an oral hygiene program would have been implemented until better oral health could be achieved.

FURTHER INVESTIGATIONS AND ASSESSMENT TOOLS

Oral–Motor Skills

There are many assessments designed to evaluate oral–motor skills involved with eating and drinking and articulation. For clinical purposes, oral–motor skills are assessed on scales such as adequate and inadequate, but for research purposes a more rigorous approach is demanded.

Eating and Drinking Skills

The *Schedule for Oral Motor Assessment* may be particularly useful for young children with mild disabilities (Reilly, Skuse, & Wolke, 2000). The *Multidisciplinary Feeding Profile* (Kenny, Koheil, et al., 1989) is useful for older children, particularly those who are dependent eaters. This test covers six domains of oral function: physical neurological, oral–facial structure, oral–facial sensory input, oral–facial motor function, ventilation phonation, and functional feeding assessment.

Alternatively, for an assessment to evaluate eating and drinking skills, the Functional Feeding Assessment–Modified (Gisel, 1994) is useful because it scores abnormal and normal behavior in the areas of spoon feeding, biting, chewing, cup drinking, straw drinking, swallowing, and drooling. The latter assessment is particularly useful when looking for a tool to demonstrate change after intervention.

Articulation

There are many tests that assess articulation and any speech–language pathologist should be able to provide this service. The Frenchay dysarthria assessment (Enderby, 1983) is particularly useful for someone with dysarthria. It also includes a section on assessing secretions.

Oral Sensation and Perception

The role of sensation inside and outside the mouth is an associated factor in poor saliva control (Weiss-Lambrou, Tétreault, & Dudley, 1989). The inability to feel food or saliva leads to spillage. Oral sensation can include touch, pressure, two-point discrimination, oral stereognosis, taste, and temperature. Unfortunately many of the assessments in this area require a cooperative client who is cognitively able (McDonald & Aungst, 1967). Currently researchers rely on parents' and clients' reports and their own observations.

The McDonald and Aungst (1967) test of oral stereognosis is "abbreviated" (the original was a longer 25-item test). It was validated on typical primary-school children. Thus there is no reliability or validity for children with a disability. However, it might prove useful. The test consists of five, three-dimensional forms. The child is blindfolded, and one of the forms is placed in the mouth. The item is then taken away and the blindfold removed. The child is then asked to identify the shape by pointing to one of five photographs.

The Ringel, Burk, and Scott (1970) test of oral stereognosis consists of 10 plastic forms in various geometric shapes. These forms are paired together, and a total of 55 pairs is generated. The individual is blindfolded, and one of the forms is placed in the mouth. The form is then removed, and another (of the pair) is placed in the mouth. This form is then removed, and the individual is asked if the two shapes were the same or different.

Oral–Motor Planning

Some people with no apparent physical limitation might have motor-planning problems. These problems may be mild (e.g., affecting the individual's sporting ability) or severe (e.g., the individual is unable to tie shoelaces). Motor-planning problems that affect the oral area are referred to as oral dyspraxia; it may occur alone but it often occurs concomitantly with muscle weakness (dysarthria). Poor oral–motor planning can result in poor speech and drooling. Clinicians frequently use the ability to copy oral movements as a diagnostic test. A subtest of the *Multidisciplinary Feeding Profile* (Kenny et al., 1989b) examines some of these skills. However, for research we recommend you use the Oral Praxis subtest of the *Southern California Sensory Integration Test* (Ayres, 1979).

Measuring the Frequency of Swallowing

A number of methods have been used to measure swallowing frequency: pharyngeal manometry (Kapila, Dodds, Helm, & Hogan, 1984), electromyography (Sochaniwskyj, Koheil, Bablich, Milner, & Kenny, 1986), ultrasound (Sonies, 1993), cervical auscultation (Lambert & Gisel, 1996; Selley et al., 2000), and observation (Barton, Leigh, & Myrvang, 1977; Murray, Langmore, Ginsberg, & Dostie, 1996). Ultrasound and cervical auscultation are the methods with the most potential clinically for a diverse population.

Pharyngeal Manometry

This technique requires the participant to pass a catheter through the nose into the pharynx. Pressure changes from pharyngeal peristalsis are recorded by using water-filled catheters. This technique is invasive, outdated, and not in current clinical use. Kapila et al. (1984) used this technique to measure swallowing rate.

Electromyography

This technique is in current use and studies the activity of muscles during a movement. Sochaniwskyj (1982) placed electrodes over the masseter, orbicularis oris, and infrahyoid muscles to study the frequency of swallowing. The movements of the muscles were recorded on a graph that describes the amplitude of a movement (peaks with specific parameters represent a swallow). Participants wearing electrodes need to be able to stay still and tolerate electrode placement.

Ultrasound

This technique was pioneered by Barbara Sonies, and although it has been used elsewhere by other researchers (Kenny, Casas, & McPherson, 1989), it does not appear to be a clinical tool. It may not be a clinical tool because of the level of skill needed to interpret the images. It is a safe, noninvasive technique that can be applied to a child or adult when standing, sitting, or lying down. The ultrasound transducer is placed beneath the individual's chin and a dynamic image of the swallowing process can be seen on the screen. This process can be done repeatedly, and audio and video recordings can be made. It has potential for measuring and visualizing the swallowing of saliva among individuals with different disabilities.

Cervical Auscultation

A clicking sound can be heard when an individual swallows. This sound has been described as two or three clicks depending on whether it is a dry or wet swallow (Cicchero, 1996). These sounds are best heard through a stethoscope, microphone, or accelerometer. The best location for placing the stethoscope has been studied extensively (Takahashi, Groher, & Micchi, 1994). Takahashi et al. recommended that the sensor be placed centrally just below the cricoid cartilage. This procedure is noninvasive, but the assessor needs to receive training to interpret the swallowing sounds. Recent developments suggest that the process might be automated, thus providing easily gathered information on swallowing rate (see Chapter 7). Cervical auscultation can be used on any participant who can tolerate a stethoscope on the neck for a short amount of time.

Measures of Drooling

There has been an ongoing search for clinically valid and useful tools. Often drooling is measured by self- or caregiver report. Drooling has been measured in a number of ways:

1. Drooling can be measured by using a collection unit, for example, a bib. Researchers have used these methods with radioactive isotopes (Ekedahl & Hallen, 1973), suction bags (Sochaniwskyj, 1982), and urine bags (Wilkie, 1970). Researchers have attempted to measure a person's daily drooling to investigate the total amount of fluid loss. However, these collection methods are highly invasive and suitable for a limited range of clients. Researchers have used weighing bibs, and although concurrent validity can be achieved (Johnson, 1990), the process may be inappropriate for age and prone to complications such as evaporation and drinks being spilled on the bibs.

2. Subjective reporting, for example, personal opinion, rating scales (see Drooling Rating Scale, Appendix A), and questionnaires (Camp-Bruno, Winsberg, Green-Parsons, & Abrams, 1989; Thomas-Stonell & Greenberg, 1988), is commonly used but is especially vulnerable to bias and misinterpretation. Blasco (1996) suggested that two different types of measurements be used to account for quantity and frequency; however, no further work has been published in this area.

3. The frequency of drooling can be measured by counting. Drooling is reported to vary from day to day and hour to hour, and obtaining an accurate representative measure requires long periods of observation. Some types of drooling are very difficult to count. Those people with long stringy drools have a much greater quantity than those people with small drips, yet the results do not show this. It is important that a qualitative aspect is included in this quantitative method. It is also impossible to count the frequency of drooling accurately when someone is aware that he or she is being measured. It can be difficult to achieve measurements from the raters if a number of measures at different times of day are required. It seems unlikely that counting the number of times a person drools will ever be able to provide researchers with a reliable, valid, and representative measure.

There is a need for researchers to provide better drooling measures. Work currently undertaken by Allaire and Brown includes assessment and measurement tools and looks promising (see Chapter 7).

The Assessment of Saliva Secretions

The assessment of saliva secretions and the assessment of drooling sometimes necessitate different approaches. The methods of drooling measurement used in this book are adapted from the work of Thomas-Stonell and Greenberg (1988). Generally, problems with saliva consistencies occur in people who have acquired or have progressive disabilities. These people may or may not have a drooling problem. (The assessment of this area is covered in the following Assessment of Secretions section.) Drooling in the developmental area—for example, people with cerebral palsy or intellectual disability—less commonly involves problems with saliva consistency (unless the condition commences after surgical intervention for drooling).

Assessment of Secretions

For some people, the loss of saliva may not be the only difficulty or even the major difficulty. Difficulty managing secretions needs careful evaluation.

Asking the individual with a salivary problem or, if appropriate, the caregiver, to fill in an oral secretion assessment form is a good place to start (see Appendix A). This provides information about the presence, consistency, amount, and timing of secretions. This information can form the basis for management decisions. The measurements are spaced at intervals during the day and are taken before and after food or drink so that the effects of these items can be noted. In some cases, it may be useful to monitor what food and fluid is taken and if there is something in particular that causes an increase in the amount of saliva or changes its consistency.

Assessment is subjective, and the qualifications of "excessive" and "very excessive" require discussion with the person filling in the form. The clinician needs to observe the problem and gain an idea of how it is perceived by the measurer.

When base measures have been taken, the treating clinician, in consultation with the team, can make decisions about whether drying or thinning saliva is the best course. After the person with the salivary problem has been stabilized on a specific medication, a reevaluation of the salivary problem will assist in determining the effectiveness of the medication. Clinical experience has shown that there is a tendency for the mouth to be dry in the morning and for the amount of secretions to increase during the day, especially after meals. The drooling problem usually peaks in late afternoon. This is in line with the Dawes and Ong (1973) findings regarding circadian rhythms.

Viscosity and Flow of Saliva

Measuring the viscosity before and after intervention may

- assist in determining which glands are producing the saliva;
- monitor the effect of specific medications on the saliva; and
- assist in evaluating one of the effects of surgical intervention.

The viscosity of the saliva can be measured by using a viscometer. To measure the viscosity, whole saliva is collected by draining, spitting, suctioning, or using the swab method (Navazesh & Christensen, 1982). Because of the difficulties of access to some people's mouths, suctioning may be the preferred method. Suctioning will not be possible with every client.

Scintigraphy or technetium scanning also has proved useful in identifying the function of glands after surgery (Hotaling, Madgy, Kuhns, Filipek, & Belenky, 1992) and may assist researchers to understand the varying results they see. The procedure for technetium scanning requires an intravenous injection and the ability to lie still for approximately an hour. This procedure is relatively expensive and requires a physician trained in nuclear medicine. Researchers' experience with this method is limited. Secretions can be observed during an oral-health assessment, which is an important part of saliva and drooling assessment.

USE OF THE ORAL SECRETION ASSESSMENT FORM

The purpose of the Oral Secretion Assessment form in Appendix A is to profile the nature of any problems with saliva in order to plan and evaluate intervention. This form allows for changes in the quantity and type of saliva, related to the time of day and the effects of eating and drinking on saliva production, to be recorded. The pattern of peaks and troughs of the saliva problems during a day will provide information for deciding the method and character of the intervention. The descriptions of the nature of the secretions also provide the clinician with information concerning the probable source of the saliva. For example, "excessive watery" saliva is most likely to occur around mealtimes and be the result of parotid secretions, or "very excessive dry mouth" is more likely to occur in the morning after mouth breathing during the night. This type of description will provide information for intervention decisions. For a clinician to gain a representative perspective of the patient's salivary problems, the patient or caregiver should fill in the assessment form for 3 days in 1 week. The clinician can convert the descriptive ratings to quantitative information by adding the values in parentheses following each descriptor in the rating system key. To calculate a severity score, the clinician can sum the ratings and then divide that number by the number of ratings for the 3 days. When the form is used in this way, the clinician can assess the effectiveness of interventions. It is recommended that clinicians use the form before and after instigating intervention.

ORAL-HEALTH ASSESSMENT

Oral health is a frequently overlooked aspect of general health. Poor oral health can influence physical functions, such as eating and drinking, saliva control, and speaking, and psychosocial function, such as social interaction, quality of life, and self-esteem. An oral-health assessment or screening and a regular oral-hygiene procedure should be included as an essential aspect of care.

This assessment is integral to a complete oral–motor assessment, parts of which are included in the *Multidisciplinary Feeding Profile* (Kenny, Koheil, et al., 1989). Measuring the presence or absence of gingivitis and the presence or absence of caries will increase researchers' knowledge of the associated effects of long-term pharmacological or surgical interventions.

Regular oral-health screening is particularly important for people who are dependent on others for care, such as people with physical or cognitive disabilities or elderly people living in residential facilities. For some people, visits to the dentist will not be possible because of access difficulties or the individual's inability to cope with the environment or the dental procedure. In these cases, oral-health screening may be the only way oral health can be assessed and monitored.

Before You Begin

Some background information on a person's experience with dentists and dental treatment may provide some valuable insights into how to approach the assessment, why an individual reacts in a particular way to having his or her mouth assessed, and some likely causes of dental problems. It also might highlight areas of specific importance to observe during the assessment. A tester should ask an individual questions about frequency of dental visits; past and present dental problems; oral or facial surgery; dental hygiene routine; eating, drinking, and speaking difficulties; and diet.

Getting Ready

The first step in undertaking an oral-health screening is to establish a relationship with the person being assessed. This relationship will help to allay anxiety associated with having someone looking in and touching the mouth and will help to reduce facial tension. It can be helpful to have the assistance of someone known to the person if he or she is apprehensive. The screening can be conducted just about anywhere. For children and people with cognitive impairment, it is probably best to conduct the screening in a familiar and comfortable environment and at a time of day when the person is likely to be most cooperative.

It is important to note that people with disabilities may have a long history of various medical and surgical procedures and may have difficulty cooperating during oral-health screening. Reassurance, empathy, and understanding will help the person relax, and involving him or her in the screening also can be useful. Explain what is going to happen in terms that the person can understand. Positioning a mirror so that he or she can see inside his or her mouth while the assessment is done may help maintain his or her interest and cooperation. It is not necessary to complete the screening all at once. In some circumstances, it may be best to complete the screening in stages over a couple of days.

The Screening Procedure

The Bethlehem Hospital and Department of Human Services *Oral Health Screening Tool* (Foulsum, 2002) is a package that includes a standardized assessment tool and an instruction booklet that allows for screening of 11 oral-health parameters: lips; tongue; saliva; inside of cheeks, roof of mouth, under tongue; gums; teeth; dentures; pain; oral-hygiene independence; bad breath; and assessment difficulties.

The instruction booklet provides background information and a step-by-step guide to oral screening. It also provides information regarding equipment requirements and infection-control procedures necessary to undertake adequate and safe oral screening. Once the tester becomes familiar with the procedure, using the instruction booklet for the first few screenings, ratings can be given using the brief rating guide listed on the form. The instruction booklet can then be used simply as a reference for clarification purposes. Each parameter is rated on a 4-point scale: *normal, mild, moderate,* and *severe*.

No direct training is required for a tester to use the *Oral Health Screening Tool*, and screening can be completed in 5 to 10 minutes by competent testers. Once the screening is complete, the tester uses the ratings to determine whether current oral-hygiene practices are adequate, changes are required to improve oral-hygiene practice, or a referral to a health professional is required. A referral guide is included in the instruction booklet to help determine when and to whom a person should be referred.

THE ASSESSMENT OF ASPIRATION OF SALIVA IN TRACHEOSTOMIZED PATIENTS

Aspiration is a frequent complication of tracheostomy (Elpern, Scott, Petro, & Ries, 1994). There are several causes of aspiration, including fixation of the trachea leading to reduced laryngeal elevation. Desensitization of the larynx and subsequent loss of protective reflexes and esophageal obstruction caused by the cuff pressing into the lower pharyngeal and upper esophageal region also lead to aspiration. Assessment of aspiration is best detected using videofluoroscopic techniques; however, a screening assessment—the blue dye test—can be used at the bedside. This assessment entails a tracheostimized patient being given a small amount of puree or fluid mixed with blue food coloring. The assessment food or fluid requires the addition of only a small amount of blue dye. It should not cause the oral structures to turn blue on contact. Blue food dye is used because it is not a biological or common food color, and therefore it is reasonable to assume the source of blue expectorated or suctioned material. After the patient has swallowed the blue bolus, the clinician checks for the following signs of aspiration:

- blue material is coughed out through the tracheostomy tube or
- blue material is suctioned from the tracheostomy tube.

During this assessment, an important factor to consider is whether the cuff on the tracheostomy tube was inflated. Blue-colored material observed in the tracheostomy tube when the cuff was inflated during the test swallows suggests that the cuff does not fit the trachea properly, that the cuff is not properly inflated, or that the cuff is leaking and that aspiration has occurred. Observation of blue material in the tracheostomy tube after the cuff has been deflated indicates that material is entering the laryngeal region, which may be caused by incomplete laryngeal elevation. Material in the tracheostomy tube after swallowing with the cuff deflated is consistent with aspiration. If blue material is observed in the tracheostomy tube immediately after the test bolus was swallowed, it is not safe for the patient to have oral intake. The presence of slight blue discoloration of tracheal secretions sometime after the assessment does not necessarily indicate that the patient is aspirating, because small amounts of secretions enter the airway and are usually expectorated or swallowed (Logeman, 1998).

REFERENCES

Ayres, A. (1979). *Southern California Sensory Integration Test.* Los Angeles: Western Psychological Services.

Barton, E. S., Leigh, E. B., & Myrvang, G. (1977). The modification of drooling behaviour in the severely retarded spastic patient. *British Journal of Mental Subnormality, 24*(47), 100–108.

Blasco, P. A. (1996). Drooling. In P. B. Sullivan & L. Rosenbloom (Eds.), *Feeding the disabled child* (pp. 92–105). London: Mac Keith.

Camp-Bruno, J. A., Winsberg, B. G., Green-Parsons, A. R., & Abrams, J. P. (1989). Efficacy of benztropine therapy for drooling. *Developmental Medicine and Child Neurology, 31*(3), 309–319.

Cicchero, J. (1996, Spring). Cervical auscultation: An assessment of the sounds of swallowing. *Australian Communication Quarterly,* 22–24.

Dawes, C., & Ong, B. Y. (1973). Circadian rhythms in the flow rate and proportional composition of parotid to whole saliva volume in man. *Archives of Oral Biology, 18,* 1145–1153.

Ekedahl, C., & Hallen, O. (1973). Quantitative measurement of drooling. *Acta Oto-laryngologica, 77,* 464–469.

Elpern, E. H., Scott, M. G., Petro, L., & Ries, M. H. (1994). Pulmonary aspiration in mechanically ventilated patients with tracheostomies. *Chest, 105*(2), 563–566.

Enderby, P. (1983). *Frenchay dysarthria assessment.* San Diego, CA: College Hill Press.

Foulsum, M. (2002). *Oral health screening tool.* Unpublished manuscript, Department of Human Services and Bethlehem Health Care, Melbourne, Australia.

Gisel, E. G. (1994). Oral motor skills following sensorimotor intervention in children with severe spastic cerebral palsy. *Dysphagia, 9*(3), 180–192.

Gisel, E. G., Schwartz, S., Petryk, A., Clarke, D., & Haberfellner, H. (2000). "Whole body" mobility after one year of intraoral appliance therapy in children with cerebral palsy and moderate eating impairment. *Dysphagia, 15*(4), 226–235.

Hotaling, A. J., Madgy, D. N., Kuhns, L. R., Filipek, L., & Belenky, W. M. (1992). Postoperative technetium scanning in patients with submandibular duct diversion. *Archives of Otolaryngology—Head and Neck Surgery, 118*(12), 1331–1333.

Johnson, H. (1990). *An exploratory study in drooling using a frequency method of measurement in a naturalistic setting.* Unpublished master's thesis, La Trobe University, Melbourne, Australia.

Kapila, Y. V., Dodds, W. J., Helm, J. F., & Hogan W. J. (1984). Relationship between swallow rate and salivary flow. *Digestive Diseases and Sciences, 29*(6), 528–533.

Kenny, D., Casas, M. J., & McPherson, K. A. (1989). Correlation of ultrasound imaging of oral swallow with ventilatory alterations in cerebral palsied and normal children: Preliminary observations. *Dysphagia, 4,* 112–117.

Kenny, D. J., Koheil, R. M., Greenberg, J., Reid, D., Milner, M., Moran, R., & Judd, P. L. (1989). Development of a multidisciplinary feeding profile for children who are dependent feeders. *Dysphagia, 4,* 16–28.

Lambert, H. C., & Gisel, E. (1996). The assessment of oral, pharyngeal and esophageal dysphagia in elderly persons. *Physical & Occupational Therapy in Geriatrics, 14*(4), 1–25.

Logeman, J. (1998). *Evaluation and treatment of swallowing disorders* (2nd ed.). Austin, TX: PRO-ED.

McDonald, E. T., & Aungst, L. F. (1967). Studies in oral sensorimotor function. In J. F. Bosma (Ed.), *Symposium on oral sensation & perception* (pp. 202–220). Springfield, IL: Thomas.

Murray, J., Langmore, S. E., Ginsberg, S., & Dostie, A. (1996). The significance of accumulated oropharyngeal secretions and swallowing frequency in predicting aspiration. *Dysphagia, 11*(2), 99–103.

Navazesh, M., & Christensen, C. M. (1982). A comparison of whole mouth resting and stimulated salivary measurement procedures. *Journal of Dental Research, 61*(10), 1158–1162.

Perry, A., Reilly, S., Bloomberg, K., & Johnson, H. (2002). *An analysis of needs for people with a disability who have complex communication needs.* Melbourne, Australia: La Trobe University.

Reddihough, D., Johnson, H., & Ferguson, E. (1992). The role of a saliva control clinic in the management of drooling. *Journal of Paediatrics and Child Health, 28*(5), 395–397.

Reilly, S., Skuse, D., & Wolke, D. (2000). *Schedule for oral motor assessment.* London: Whurr.

Ringle, R. L., Burk, K. W., & Scott, C. M. (1970). Tactile perception: Form discrimination in the mouth. In J. F. Bosma (Ed.), *Second Symposium on Oral Sensation & Perception* (pp. 410–415). Springfield, IL: Thomas.

Selley, W. G., Parrott, L. C., Lethbridge, P. C., Flack, R. C., Ellis, R. E., Johnston, K. J., & Tripp, J. H. (2000). Noninvasive techniques for assessment and management planning of oral-pharyngeal dysphagia in children with cerebral palsy. *Developmental Medicine and Child Neurology, 42,* 617–623.

Sochaniwskyj, A. E. (1982). Drool quantification: Noninvasive technique. *Archives of Physical Medicine and Rehabilitation, 63*(12), 605–607.

Sochaniwskyj, A. E., Koheil, R. M., Bablich, K., Milner, K., & Kenny, D. J. (1986). Oral motor functioning, frequency of swallowing and drooling in normal children and in children with cerebral palsy. *Archives of Physical Medicine and Rehabilitation, 67,* 866–874.

Sonies, B. C. (1993). Dysphagia diagnostics and Donner: Experiences in the decade of change. *Dysphagia, 8*(3), 166–169.

Takahashi, K., Groher, M. E., & Micchi, K. (1994). Symmetry and reproducibility of swallowing sounds. *Dysphagia, 9,* 168–173.

Thomas-Stonell, N., & Greenberg, J. (1988). Three treatment approaches and clinical factors in the reduction of drooling. *Dysphagia, 3*(2), 73–78.

Weiss-Lambrou, R., Tétreault, S., & Dudley, J. (1989). The relationship between oral sensation and drooling in persons with cerebral palsy. *American Journal of Occupational Therapy, 43*(3), 155–161.

Wilkie, T. F. (1970). The surgical treatment of drooling: A follow-up report of five years. *Journal of Plastic and Reconstructive Surgery, 45*(6), 549–554.

CHAPTER

Maintaining Oral Health

Learning Outcomes

- *Understand how diet affects oral health*

- *Become familiar with a range of aids for oral hygiene*

- *Learn how to clean teeth and gums*

- *Learn about the application of fluoride*

- *Learn how to assist teeth cleaning with someone who is orally oversensitive to touch*

PREVENTION OF ORAL-HEALTH DISEASE

There are four aspects to preventing oral disease.

1. *Diet.* It is important to reduce the frequency of intake as well as the total amount of sugary foods and drinks. This can be difficult for individuals with disabilities because the choice of food is often limited or controlled by other parties, for example, day centers, group homes, and so forth. Drinks are often not considered as part of a dietary analysis; however, most soft drinks (carbonated and otherwise) have a very high sugar content and increase the possibility of caries. Increasing water intake will not only serve to reduce the amount of sugary drinks consumed but also will help to maintain hydration and optimize the production of saliva with all its protective actions.

Milk and milk-based drinks such as milk shakes tend to adhere to the teeth, particularly for those individuals with dysphagia, low motor muscle tone, and other such oral–motor problems in which oral clearance is poor. The prolonged exposure of hard dental tissue to milk (including milk shakes, which have added sugar content), particularly in the absence of normal salivary flow, will predispose an individual to dental decay. Such high caries risk is commonly seen in infants who are exposed to prolonged, on-demand bottle-feeding practices and who subsequently go on to develop early childhood caries (Seow, 1998). Encouraging the use of water as the last fluid intake after a meal, just before bedtime and, in the case of infants, in the bottle at night, will provide an opportunity for the oral cavity to return to a neutral pH and therefore reduce the caries risk.

2. *Oral hygiene.* Effective tooth brushing will help remove plaque and acid-producing bacteria from the mouth, which is essential to reduce the severity of gingivitis and help prevent periodontitis. Effective plaque removal can be achieved relatively simply using a manual toothbrush; however, some individuals with disabilities find this quite difficult. The use of an electric toothbrush can be very beneficial in those circumstances in which individuals have limited manual dexterity, coordination, or concentration. Many caregivers find it easier (and quicker) to use an electric toothbrush with the person with a disability. A problem often encountered in individuals with disabilities is that they may be unable to coordinate muscle control adequately for a caregiver or parent to perform effective brushing. A number of specifically designed aids are now available for use in different situations. The equipment section in this chapter provides some examples of these oral-hygiene aids. Other methods for mechanically removing plaque include dental floss and interdental brushes, however these techniques require a high degree of manual dexterity and should be done in conjunction with the advice and training of a qualified oral-health professional.

Chemical mouthwashes can be used to help control plaque. Professional supervision is advisable when using these products. For example, chlorhexidine has a broad spectrum of bactericidal activity against bacteria such as the mutans streptococci. When used as a mouthwash, chlorhexidine has been shown to prevent the buildup of dental plaque (Löe & Schiött, 1970). There is little evidence that these mouthwashes have any effect on established plaque and so should be used in conjunction with effective mechanical cleaning. It should be noted, however, that long-term use of chlorhexidine is associated with changes in taste sensation, irritation of the mucosa (particularly with those preparations that are alcohol based), and can stain teeth and some filling materials. For people with disabilities and other special needs, the use of chlorhexidine in conjunction with mechanical brushing under professional supervision can significantly reduce chronic gingivitis (Francis, Hunter, & Addy, 1987).

3. *Fluoride.* Fluoride enhances the ability of teeth to resist demineralization caused by the acids produced in dental plaque. Apart from systemic water fluoridation (which is beyond the control of the individual), the most common source of fluoride is that available in commercial toothpastes. Most adult toothpastes containing around 1,000 ppm (parts per million) are known to be effective in reducing caries (Murray & Naylor, 1996). Children younger than the age of 6 years should be encouraged to use a lower strength fluoride toothpaste (400 ppm) and to brush under parental supervision to prevent ingestion of large amounts of toothpaste. Long-term ingestion of excessive amounts of fluoride during the period when teeth are developing results in dental fluorosis. Clinically, fluorosis has a wide variety of presentations, from small white flecking on the crowns of the teeth to moderately sized opaque white patches and, in the most severe scenario, arrested tooth development, leaving the crowns pitted, brown, and defective. However, the latter presentations are rare and are essentially seen only in individuals who spent their developing years in regions where excessively high concentrations of fluoride existed naturally in the water supply (e.g., Somalia). However, caution should be exercised in areas where the water supplies are optimally fluoridated (0.5 to 1.0 mg/L) when advising on which toothpaste to use and certainly when considering additional fluoride supplementation, particularly in relation to children.

The use of additional topical fluoride supplements can be of significant benefit on an individual basis, particularly for people who are at high risk of dental decay. This would include people with special needs, those with high sugar intake, those who have had salivary gland surgery, and people for whom there is a significant change not only in the amount of saliva but also in its composition.

There can be significant advantages gained from using fluoride mouthwashes or topical gels on a regular basis at home. When compliance is uncertain, topical fluoride applied regularly by an oral-health professional can be equally beneficial. There is a wide range of topical fluoride preparations available worldwide. All fluoride mouthwashes and gels should be used on the advice of a qualified oral-health professional.

4. *Regular dental checkups.* As mentioned previously, many strategies used to prevent oral disease, be it decay or gum disease, are most effectively done in conjunction with the advice and supervision of an oral-health professional. The appropriate dose, frequency, and techniques of chemical and physical methods of preventing oral disease are optimized by discussing the individual case with an oral-health professional. For people with special needs, dental care can often pose a challenge as there still exist significant barriers to accessing appropriate, experienced care. The International Association for Disability and Oral Health (www.iadh.org) is committed to improving access to and the quality of oral health for people with disabilities. The British Society for Disability and Oral Health (www.bsdh.org.uk) also provides useful information for those interested in this area.

ORAL-HYGIENE EQUIPMENT

There is a range of toothbrushes, toothpastes, flosses, and mouthwashes available for helping with oral hygiene.

Toothbrushes

The major distinction between toothbrushes is that they are either *manual* or *electric*.

Manual Toothbrushes

Traditional toothbrushes require good manual dexterity. In general, a small head enables the best access to teeth and gums, particularly in the back of the mouth, and more precision when brushing. Soft bristles are gentler on the gums and help reduce the abrasive effects of brushing on the surface of the teeth. If necessary, soaking the brush in hot water will further soften bristles; however, this practice should be limited to those people who have specific conditions that result in a very sensitive oral mucosa (e.g., people undergoing acute chemotherapy or people with epidermolysis bullosa).

Although a large variety of toothbrushes is available, some people may find that adapting the shape of the toothbrush will help make cleaning easier. To adapt the shape, heat the plastic handle of the toothbrush in a cup of hot water and mold it into the desired shape. Wrapping a foam bandage around the handle also can facilitate more effective brushing for people with limited manual dexterity (see Figure 4.1). Some toothbrushes, such as the Collis-Curve, have curved bristles that enable simultaneous brushing of the inside and outside surfaces of the teeth. These brushes are popular with people with disabilities (see Figure 4.2).

Electric Toothbrushes

Electric toothbrushes can be very helpful for people with disabilities. They enable easy access to teeth and gums because they have a small brush head and clean more rapidly. The cordless type is more portable and is generally preferable. Some people are very sensitive to the vibration of electric toothbrushes, because it may stimulate an undesirable increase in muscle tone. Electric toothbrushes are unsuitable for this group. Some individuals may have a strong aversion to the vibratory sensation in their mouth caused by the electric toothbrush. This may be caused by hypersensitivity, and an oral desensitization program may help to make the use of an electric toothbrush more tolerable. Some

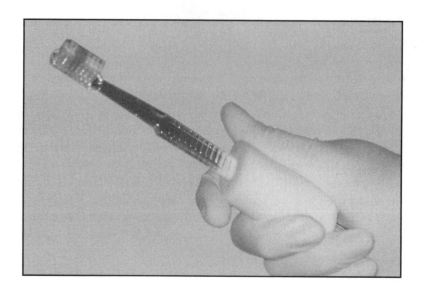

FIGURE 4.1.
Slide bandage
around toothbrush.

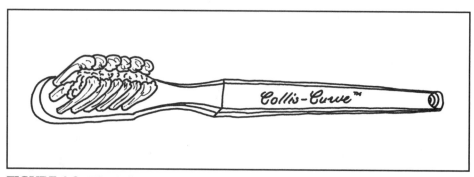

FIGURE 4.2. The Collis-Curve toothbrush. *Note.* From www.colliscurve.com. Reprinted with permission of Collis Curve USA.

people find the initial vibration frightening, but if the toothbrush is introduced slowly there is more success. If a person still exhibits distress after an oral desensitization program, then an electric toothbrush will be inappropriate.

Suction toothbrushes are a useful dental hygiene tool for people who have difficulty spitting out pooled saliva and cleaning agents (see Figure 4.3). The Suction Oral Swab made by Sage Products, Inc., provides a single-use suction sponge tip or sponge-brush combined tip that attaches to a standard suction apparatus. This innovative device allows the caregiver to clean the person's teeth and suction away oral pooling intermittently throughout the procedure.

Toothbrushes of any type may be inappropriate for some people, for example, people on chemotherapy who have very low blood counts and individuals with fragile mucosal conditions. In these circumstances, using disposable foam swabs such as Toothettes or jumbo cotton swabs to clean around the mouth can be a useful alternative (see Figure 4.4). These swabs will not be as effective as brushing to remove plaque; however, they can help to maintain oral health until toothbrushing is recommended. Lemon glycerine swabs should be avoided because the glycerine dries out the oral mucosa, and the lemon is irritating to mucosa and its acidity can increase the possibility of caries.

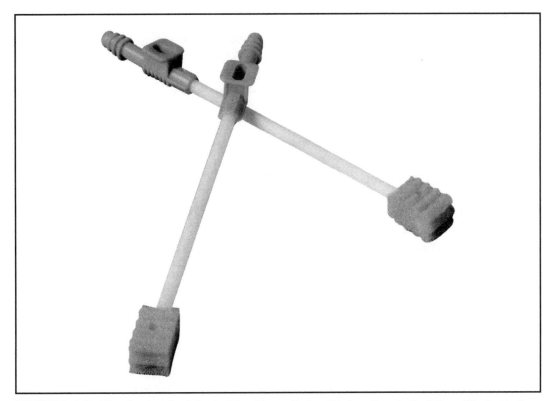

FIGURE 4.3. The Suction Oral Swab. *Note.* From *Patient Hygiene: Part 1; Oral Care: The Inside Story* (p. 16). Copyright by Sage Products. Reprinted with permission.

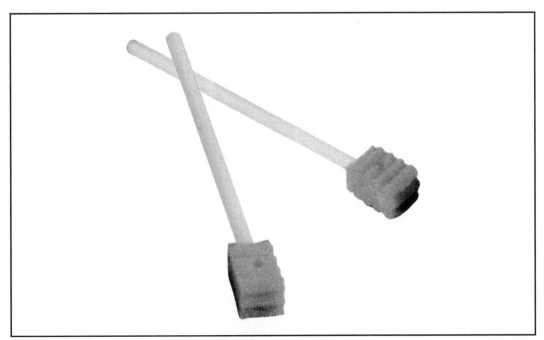

FIGURE 4.4. Toothettes. *Note.* From *Patient Hygiene: Part 1; Oral Care: The Inside Story* (p. 16). Copyright by Sage Products. Reprinted with permission.

Toothpastes

The choice of toothpaste tends to depend on personal preference. Some people will prefer a bland taste, and others will prefer a strong taste. However, it is important to use a toothpaste that contains fluoride. Although more than 95% of toothpastes contain fluoride, there are a few commercially available nonfluoridated pastes, and these are not recommended. Children younger than the age of 6 years should use a low-fluoride toothpaste (see previous discussion on fluoride). Some individuals may dislike a change in brand of toothpaste, which may result in noncompliance with the oral-hygiene procedure. Gradually introducing very small amounts of the new toothpaste or reverting to the usual brand may be all that is required to overcome the problem.

When abrasion of the tooth surface has resulted in sensitivity to hot or cold temperatures or to touch, using a toothpaste specifically designed for sensitive teeth will help to remineralize the tooth surface over time and will reduce sensitivity. Low-foaming toothpastes are available and may be preferable for people with secretion management and swallowing problems.

Floss

Dental floss is used to clean the space between teeth and between the tooth and gum surface. Floss is available in waxed (soluble), unwaxed, string, ribbon, flavored, and unflavored varities. When manual dexterity is impaired, floss can be used with a floss holder. Effective flossing can be difficult and practice is required when self-flossing or flossing another person's teeth. Advice should be sought from an oral-health professional prior to commencing flossing.

NORMALIZING ORAL SENSATION

Before beginning an oral-hygiene routine, some individuals may need to undergo a program to normalize oral sensation. This program is helpful for people who exhibit a strong reaction to objects, textures, or tastes being introduced to the mouth. These reactions may include having pain, pulling away, or having a hypersensitive gag reflex.

The aim of the program is to gradually decrease the sensitivity of the mouth over time so that responses are diminished or inhibited and oral activities such as oral hygiene can be undertaken without distress. The following guide can be adapted to meet the needs of the individual. The steps should be commenced once daily and increased to twice then three times daily. The number of repetitions of each step will gradually increase as the individual's tolerance levels increase and sensitivity reduces. Gradually build up to completing 10 repetitions of each activity three times per day.

To begin, select a stimulus item:

> finger
> spoon
> cotton swab
> foam swab
> soft toothbrush
> electric toothbrush

Items are listed from easiest to most difficult to tolerate. The finger should only be used outside the mouth in case of biting, and care should be taken when using a spoon to avoid the possibility of damage to the teeth if the bite reflex is active. In these cases, use only soft items. Select from the list the item that the person is most able to cope with and gradually work through the steps below. Select the next item in the list when the previous item is well tolerated.

Step 1. Rub the stimulus item across the back of the hand. When this is easily tolerated, move to other parts of the body such as the neck, cheek, and eventually around the outside of the mouth. This step will be helpful for very sensitive individuals who have a strong aversion to oral activity, but it will not be required for people who have oral hypersensitivity.

Step 2. Rub the stimulus item along the inside of the lips. Use long, firm strokes starting just inside the top lip. Gradually move along each side of the upper lip. When tolerated, do the same on the lower lip.

Step 3. Using long, firm strokes, rub the stimulus item along the outside of the upper gums and teeth. Begin at the front of the mouth and gradually slide along the side going back as far as the person will tolerate. When tolerated, repeat along the lower gums.

Step 4. Beginning just behind the front teeth, rub the stimulus item back along the roof of the mouth. Stop just before the gag reflex is triggered or an aversive reaction occurs. Gradually, this point will move farther back in the mouth as the person becomes less sensitive. Begin on one side of the mouth then move to the other side and finally down the center line.

Step 5. Proceed to the tongue. Beginning at the tip, run the stimulus item down one side of the tongue to the point just before the gag reflex triggers or an aversive reaction occurs. Proceed to the other side of the tongue and finally down the center. The goal is eventually to move the item as far back as the arches (faucial pillars) before the gag reflex triggers.

Step 6. Choose the next stimulus item from the list and repeat Steps 1 through 5.

Once this program is completed, the person should be able to cope with a range of stimulus items moving comfortably around the mouth, which will assist the person's ability to cope with oral screening, oral hygiene, and dental procedures.

THE ORAL-HYGIENE ROUTINE

Ideally, teeth cleaning should be carried out after every meal; however, this is not always practical. Cleaning the teeth and gums twice a day—after breakfast and before bed—and rinsing or swabbing the mouth with water during the day after foods and flavored drinks will be beneficial. It is necessary to floss the teeth only once per day.

Positioning

When assisting another person, he or she should be seated comfortably in an upright position with his or her head level. If necessary, reduce distractions by turning off the television or seating the person away from other people. Place a towel across the chest to prevent soiling clothes. If you are a right-handed caregiver, stand behind and to the right of the person who is receiving assistance. Place your left arm around and behind the head (the head can rest on the arm as added support), support the chin and facilitate mouth opening by using your left hand. If necessary, gently insert two gloved fingers to part the lips and assist the person to open his or her mouth. You should ensure that the person is comfortably in position before beginning. Although a slight tilt of the head backward may be helpful in allowing access, try to avoid placing the head and neck in hyperextension because this may impede breathing or swallowing in individuals with orofacial muscular impairment. It is important to be tuned in to the comfort of the person throughout the oral-hygiene procedure and make necessary adjustments or have regular rests as required.

Brushing

Moisten the toothbrush and apply a small amount of toothpaste (approximately the size of a pea) to the bristles. If using a swab, moisten and apply toothpaste. If the swab is treated with a cleaning agent, follow the supplier's directions. Hold the brush or swab against the tooth and gum surfaces so that the bristles cover the margin between the teeth and gums. Using gentle pressure, brush in a small circular motion over the surfaces of the teeth and over the gum margin. Work systematically around the mouth beginning with the outside surfaces then the inside surfaces of the upper and lower teeth and gums. Finish the procedure by brushing back and forth along the biting surfaces of the upper and lower teeth. See Figure 4.5 for pictures of this procedure. Allow regular rests for spitting out, swabbing out or suctioning, rinsing, and swallowing. Some people will find it difficult to keep their mouth open for any length of time and will need rest periods of several minutes or the support of a bite block throughout the procedure.

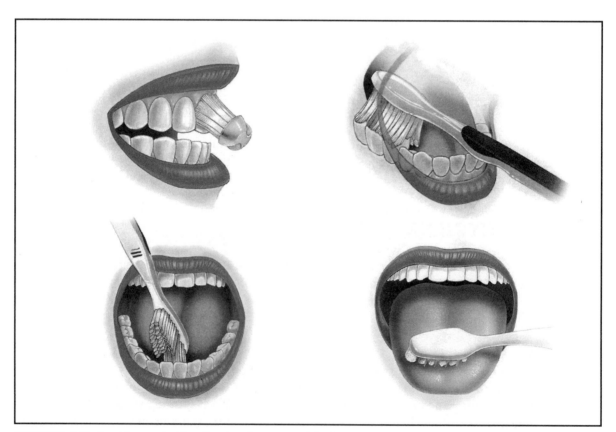

FIGURE 4.5. Brushing teeth. *Note.* Reprinted courtesy of Oral-B/Braun.

Flossing

Take a length of floss of approximately 30 cm. Begin at one end of the floss and wrap it so that there is a taut piece of floss of approximately 1.5 cm between the fingers or thumbs of each hand. Each individual will develop his or her own method of doing this. If using a floss holder, follow the manufacturer's directions to attach floss. Gently slide the floss back and forth with mild upward pressure between the contact points of the teeth. Take care not to apply too much pressure, because this may cause the floss to flick quickly and injure the gum.

When the floss has moved through the contact point and is moving freely between the teeth at the gum line, gently slide the floss under the gum where it meets the base of the tooth. Move the floss up and down two or three times to clear any debris and to stimulate blood circulation. Do this on both sides for each tooth. Gently slide the floss back and forth again through the contact point to remove. Move along the floss to a new section and continue to floss between all teeth. Remember to run the floss under the gum margin of back teeth and teeth next to spaces. See Figure 4.6 for pictures of this procedure.

When flossing is first commenced, it is common for the gums to bleed and for minor swelling along the gum margin to occur. This is a sign of gum irritation and will rapidly resolve with regular flossing and toothbrushing. Rinsing with salty water will aid healing. If there is reason for concern, a referral to a dentist is recommended.

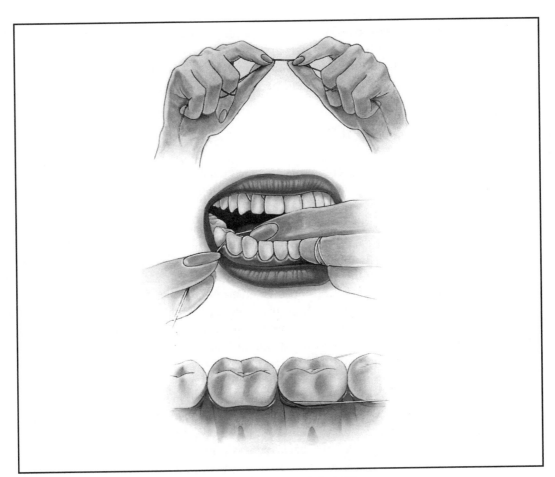

FIGURE 4.6. Flossing teeth. *Note.* Reprinted courtesy of Oral-B/Braun.

Rinsing

Rinsing the mouth two or three times after cleaning and again after flossing will remove any residue. Tepid water is appropriate if teeth and gums are sensitive to temperature. Mouthwashes should be used only according to manufacturer or dentist recommendations. Some people will have difficulty expectorating, therefore the use of moist swabs, tissues, or suction to clear the mouth after the procedure may be necessary. If the lips are dry, apply lip balm after the oral-hygiene procedure.

Dentures

Dentures should be cleaned and checked daily. Carefully remove the denture or have the person remove it. Handle dentures with care, because they are prone to cracks and breaks. If there is damage to the denture, refer the person to a dentist or dental technician. Always hold dentures over a towel when checking, and use a plastic container for cleaning. If it is absolutely necessary to clean dentures over a sink, place a washer in the bottom of the sink to protect them in case of mishap. Clean dentures using a soft toothbrush and denture cleaning agent. Carefully brush over all surfaces, including teeth and clasps, then rinse well. Before reinserting, moisten the denture so it will be more comfortable and easier to reposition. If the person does not wear the denture overnight, it should be stored in a container of water to prevent drying and cracking. If the denture is stained, a cleaning solution may be added to the container.

Oral Lubrication

For people who suffer from dry mouth, the application of an oral lubricant after oral hygiene will increase comfort. There is a range of lubricants available in spray, drop, and gel forms. Water-based products are preferable to oil-based products when there is a risk of aspiration. Oral lubricants should be applied with a gloved finger or cotton swab over the gums, across the tongue, and on the roof of the mouth.

ASSISTIVE TECHNIQUES

Some people will present with issues that make undertaking oral-hygiene procedures more difficult or uncomfortable. Some strategies can be implemented to help manage these issues.

Active Reflexes. Bite and gag reflexes can be hyperactive in some individuals, particularly those with high tone muscles, for example, spastic cerebral palsy, traumatic brain injury, and so forth. Placing a person in flexion will help to reduce hyperextension and activation of reflexes. To do this, ensure his or her bottom is positioned back in the seat, which should place the hips at an angle of 90 degrees or less. Ensure the knees and ankles are also at 90 degrees. If the person is still extending, stand in front and place the hands over the shoulders to the shoulder blades, encourage the person to look at his or her stomach, and gently bring the trunk forward. Finally, assist the head to come forward by firmly grasping the crown of the head and gently moving it into position. It should be noted that placing the hand behind the head may increase neck hyperextension. Adjusting wheelchair footplates or using cushions and rolled towels may be helpful in maintaining the flexed position. Maintain mouth opening by placing a rubber or compressed foam bite block between the back teeth on the opposite side to which you are cleaning (see Figure 4.7). If a bite block is not available, a wad of cotton wool or a soft cork wrapped in gauze can be used in the same way.

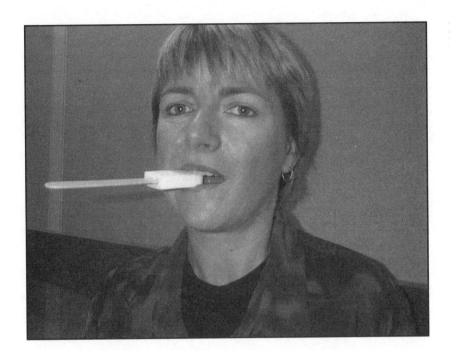

FIGURE 4.7.
Bite block.

Tongue Thrust. Some people will find it difficult to inhibit a strong tongue thrust. A flexed posture with the head slightly forward rather than extended helps. The tongue thrust will be less of a problem if the person is comfortably positioned.

Compliance. In some instances, regardless of the sensitivity and expertise of caregivers and the techniques implemented, it will be necessary to conduct oral assessment and dental treatment under general anesthetic. Sensitivity, support, and an explanation of the procedure should be given by the treating clinician prior to the day of the anaesthetic. At this time, the person and his or her family should be encouraged to ask questions and clarify information so that they have a full understanding of what will occur and what to prepare for. A follow-up appointment should be made so that results and ongoing management can be discussed.

Oral-health screening and routine oral hygiene will not necessarily eliminate all dental problems, but it is an effective strategy to help maintain quality of life and to prevent the development of dental health problems. Regular examination by a dentist should be conducted on a 6- to 12-month basis.

REFERENCES

Francis, J. R., Hunter, B., & Addy, M. (1987). A comparison of three delivery methods of chlorhexidine in handicapped children. Effects on plaque, gingivitis and tooth staining. *Journal of Periodontal Research*, *58*, 451–455.

Löe, H., & Schiött, C. R. (1970). The effect of mouthrinses and topical application of chlorhexidine on the development of dental plaque and gingivitis in man. *Journal of Periodontal Research*, *5*(2), 79–83.

Murray, J. J., & Naylor, M. N. (1996). Fluoride and dental caries. In J. Murray (Ed.), *Prevention of oral disease* (pp. 32–67). Oxford, England: Oxford University Press.

Seow, K. (1998). Biological mechanisms of early childhood caries. *Community Dentistry and Oral Epidemiology*, *26*(Suppl. 1), 8–27.

CHAPTER

Sensory–Motor Approaches to Oral–Facial Facilitation

Learning Outcomes

- *Be familiar with a range of oral-stimulation techniques*

- *Be aware of the limited evidence base for oral–facial techniques*

- *Understand the importance of gross physical preparation before oral–facial facilitation*

- *Follow a brushing and icing program designed for saliva control*

- *Follow ideas from instruction sheets to improve oral awareness and lip and tongue movements*

Many people with inadequate saliva control demonstrate limitations in oral movements, for example, lip closure or chewing. The reasons are often complex and include aspects from the sensory and motor nervous systems (see Chapters 1 and 2). Physiotherapy, occupational therapy, and speech therapy approaches have arisen from the works of Ayers (1979), Castillo-Morales (see Fischer-Brandies, Avalle, & Limbrock, 1987), and Rood (see Draper, 1968). Oral–motor facilitation has been used with success in developing mealtime skills (Gisel, 1996; Gisel, Applegate-Ferrante, Benson, & Bosma, 1996; Haberfellner, Schwartz, & Gisel, 2001). In this chapter, we suggest therapeutic techniques that are used in clinical practice for improving oral–motor skills. Many of these techniques have a limited evidence base.

The techniques of brushing and icing have been developed from a neurophysiological treatment program (Rood, 1954) based on the principle that proprioceptive stimulation can assist the development of normal movement patterns. Techniques include the use of icing, brushing, vibration, and manipulation through light and firm touch, tapping, stroking, stretching, and patting. These techniques attempt to normalize muscle tone and to provide intensive sensory input aimed at increasing oral awareness and discrimination. There is little published research using these techniques (Domaracki & Sisson, 1990; Falk, Wells, & Toth, 1976; Grant, 1982; Loiselle, 1979), yet therapists frequently use these strategies. It appears that the intensity of input affects the outcome, but there is little agreement as to the speed or intensity of vibration or massage that is desirable.

Deep massage and stimulation also have been used, often accompanied by stimulatory plates (Carlstedt, Dahllöf, Nilsson, & Modeer, 1996; Fischer-Brandies et al., 1987; Limbrock, Fischer-Brandies, & Avalle, 1991; Russell, 2001). Deep massage and stimulation also can be seen as part of a sensory program to prepare the body for movement. Sensory integration techniques (Ayers, 1979; Oetter, Richter, & Frick, 1995) aim to develop the coordination of oral sensory–motor skills (including respiration) by selecting materials that develop rhythm, frequency, intensity, and duration of oral sensory–motor activities.

Well-researched strategies for normalizing the oral sensory–motor system are still needed by parents, therapists, and dentists. However, in this chapter we expand on some of the sensory programs that have been found to be clinically useful.

BASIC POSITIONING

General posture can be improved by therapeutic sports such as horseback riding and swimming (Rantala, 2001). The principles of cephalocaudal development underlie oral treatment; thus, providing good gross motor control will assist in developing fine oral–motor control. The relationship between body and head posture, jaw control, and swallowing is complex and needs to be attended to on an individual basis. For clients with severe disabilities, the position of the wheelchair (e.g., reclining or upright) may affect their ability to swallow (Morton, Bonas, Fourie, & Minford, 1993).

Many clients extend their neck or jaw while eating, which may be a result of using an extensor pattern (Morris & Klein, 1987). There is often a concomitant pattern of shoulder-girdle fixation when the neck becomes retracted. These patterns also will affect the oral movements. When these patterns are evident, physical assistance with jaw control may be necessary. All therapeutic intervention should be applied when the person is in a controlled posture. Slight flexion is preferred to extension. Initially, full head and neck control may be required. When possible, the person should be encouraged to take control of his or her posture once he or she understands what is needed. Good posture is essential for any motor program (e.g., oral appliances, vibratory techniques).

ORAL–FACIAL FACILITATION

Oral–facial facilitation techniques have been used to improve control of saliva with people who have hypertonic (high tone, spastic) and hypotonic (low tone, flaccid) muscles. The following clinical population groups have hypertonic or hypotonic muscles: children with cerebral palsy and other neurological conditions; children with intellectual impairment, for example, Down syndrome; children with low muscle tone, usually associated with developmental delay; adults with cerebral palsy and other developmental neurological conditions; adults with acquired neurological impairment, such as stroke; and adults with a progressive neurological impairment, such as amyotrophic lateral sclerosis or multiple sclerosis.

Oral–facial facilitation techniques should be used only by people who have some knowledge of head and neck anatomy. It is important to know the names, insertions, and functions of the muscles (see Figure 5.1). Clinical experience has shown that oral–facial facilitation techniques vary in their effectiveness. It is therefore appropriate to trial these techniques before introducing them into the daily routine. It also is important to introduce these techniques gradually to build up tolerance to the sensory input, because some individuals may initially find the stimulation aversive.

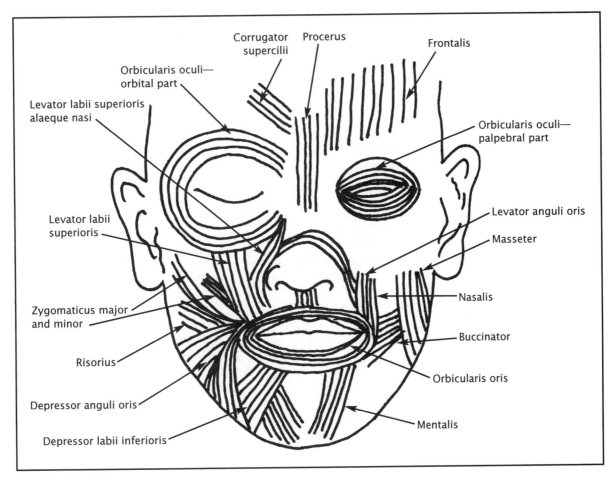

FIGURE 5.1. Facial muscles.

PHYSICAL POSITIONING

Before using any of these techniques, position the individual receiving treatment appropriately. When sitting, it is important to ensure that the shoulder girdle, trunk, and pelvis are stable and that the feet are flat on the floor or footplates of the wheelchair. The back of the neck should be straight, with the chin slightly tucked (see Figures 5.2 and 5.3). With individuals who have severe disabilities and who are confined to bed, it is important that they are in a comfortable and well-supported position, sitting up as much as possible.

Once the individual is in a stable and comfortable position, one (or a combination) of the following programs can be tried: icing, brushing, vibration, manipulation, and oral sensory–motor exercises.

ICING

The application of ice directly over the target muscle has been found to normalize muscle tone in some individuals (see Figure 5.4), thereby improving oral–motor function and enhancing sensory awareness. To maximize the effectiveness of this procedure, an oral activity such as eating or exercise should directly follow icing. The effects of icing are immediate and may last between 5 and 30 minutes (Hamer, 1972).

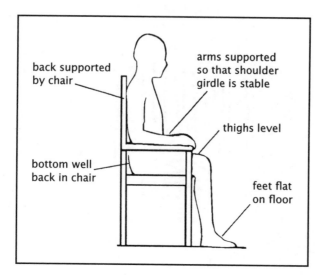

FIGURE 5.2. Correct positioning for oral–facial facilitation: stable shoulder girdle, pelvis, and trunk.

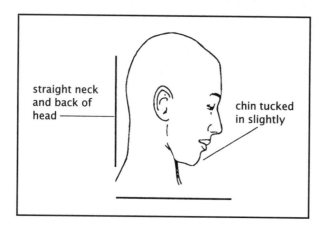

FIGURE 5.3. Head position: head and neck elongated and chin slightly tucked.

Application of Ice to the Face

- Apply firm, even pressure along the muscle in the direction of the muscle movement.

- Ice facial areas first, proceed to the mouth, and then inside the mouth.

- An ice cube can be sucked to normalize tone in the tongue, mouth, and pharynx. Ensure that there are no sharp edges (Langley, 1987).

- Ice should be applied for 3 to 10 seconds, depending on the tolerance level of the individual and the effectiveness of the procedure.

- Ice along the cheeks (buccinator muscles).

- Ice over the masseter muscles.

- Ice around the lips (orbicularis oris muscles).

It has been found that ice helps to stimulate a delayed or absent swallow reflex (Logeman, 1983).

FIGURE 5.4. Diagram for sequence and direction of icing and brushing techniques.

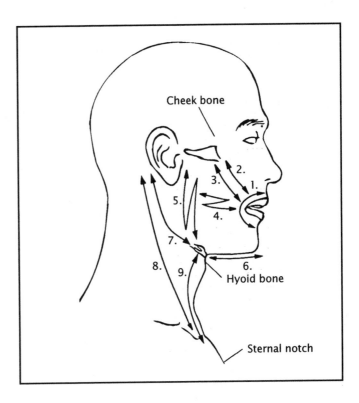

Application of Ice To Stimulate Swallow Reflex

The following are strategies that have been found to be useful:

- Apply an ice pack to the neck at the level of the thyroid cartilage.

- Apply ice directly to the thyroid notch.

- Apply ice to the anterior faucial arches (see Figure 5.5) and immediately above the uvula using a frozen wetted cotton swab or chilled laryngeal mirror (to be used only if tone is normal or low and there is no bite reflex).

When using these icing procedures, the following considerations should be taken into account:

- Ice facial areas first, proceed to the mouth, and then inside the mouth.

- Ice can be a noxious stimulus that may lead to seizures in some individuals with epilepsy or may increase spasticity and rigidity in others.

- Ice may not be effective and may cause great discomfort for individuals who are hypersensitive or who are sensory defensive.

- Ice may cause "ice burns," which are evident by reddening of the skin; therefore, care must be taken during application.

- Sucking ice is not recommended for individuals with severe tongue thrust because it reinforces the thrusting pattern (Gallender, 1979).

- Icing in the region of the carotid sinus (behind the left ear) should be avoided in individuals with severe cardiac problems.

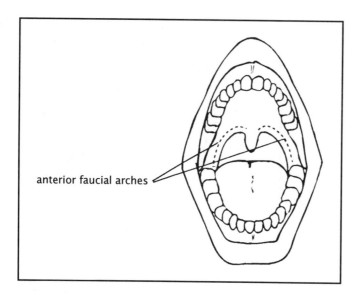

FIGURE 5.5. Anterior faucial arches.

anterior faucial arches

The following ideas for handling ice have been found useful:

- small ice cubes, made from water (because sweet or citrus fruit juice cubes increase salivation)

- iced, wetted cotton swabs made by placing swabs in individual fingers of a surgical glove and freezing (Note: Some surgical gloves have powder inside; therefore the ice will be gritty if these gloves are used.)

- crushed ice in a disposable surgical glove (the fingers can be sucked like a frozen treat)

- frozen fruit juice on a stick (molds are available in supermarkets)

- ice sticks made by freezing water frozen in a plastic straw (Push 2 cm of the ice out of the straw and apply to the desired area, holding the straw firmly [Morris & Klein, 1987].)

- a small, long-handled laryngeal mirror that has been placed in ice water (The chilled mirror is especially useful for cold stimulation to faucial arches [Logeman, 1983]. Note: Always be wary of putting objects in the mouth if the person has a strong reflexive bite.)

BRUSHING

Brushing is another procedure reported to normalize tone and increase sensory awareness. The effects of brushing are said to occur 20 to 30 minutes after the procedure (Langley, 1987). Brushing should take place a half hour before a meal or a half hour before an oral activity or exercise.

Methods for Brushing

For manual brushing, use a medium-sized camel hair paintbrush. Use light, rapid strokes along the muscle in the direction of the muscle movement. It is recommended that brushing not take place for more than 3 seconds per muscle (Langley, 1987).

For fast rotary brushing or battery-operated brushing, provide firm, even brushing to the muscle in the direction of the muscle movement. This method is considered to be more effective than manual brushing for stimulating hypotonic (flaccid) muscles.

Procedure for Brushing

Refer to Figure 5.4 for sequence and direction of brushing technique.

- Brush along the cheeks (buccinator).

- Brush the biting and inside surfaces of teeth.

- Brush tongue, lips, and cheeks to stimulate muscle tone.

- An electric toothbrush can be introduced with the above regime and may be particularly useful for asymmetrical oral–facial structures, if the individual can tolerate it.

When using these brushing procedures, take into account the following considerations:

- Introduce brushing to the face first, proceed to the mouth, and then inside the mouth.

- Do not stimulate the temporalis muscle, because this will result in jaw retraction (Gallender, 1979).

- Monitor the reaction to brushing and grade the stimulation accordingly.

VIBRATION

Vibration aims to increase proprioceptive input and facilitate more normal tone. Clinically, it has been found to be more effective than brushing, perhaps due to its more intense stimulation. Although considered to be effective for stimulating hypotonic muscles, it also has been useful for those people with hypertonic muscles.

If the individual reacts strongly to vibration applied to the oral area, develop tolerance by first applying the stimulus to other parts of the body (e.g., arms, backs of hands) for brief intervals (Grant, 1982).

Procedure for Application of Vibration (Manual and Battery Operated)

- Apply vibration directly to the target muscles in the direction of the movement for approximately 6 to 10 seconds (refer to Figure 5.4).

- Vibrate along the cheeks (buccinator muscles).

- Vibrate over the masseter muscles.

- Vibrate around the mouth (orbicularis oris muscles).

- Vibrate under the chin.

- Apply vibration directly above the thyroid notch and over the thyroid lamina to stimulate a swallow reflex and cough.

- Vibrate the area from either side of the nostrils in a downward direction to the bottom of the upper lip (see Figure 5.6) to decrease upper lip retraction (Morris & Klein, 1987).

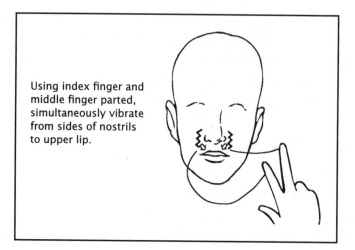

Using index finger and middle finger parted, simultaneously vibrate from sides of nostrils to upper lip.

FIGURE 5.6. Vibration between nose and upper lip.

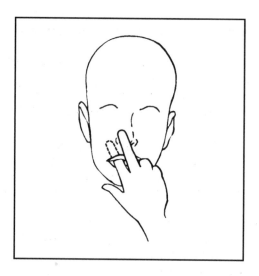

FIGURE 5.7. Vibration of the cheek using index and middle fingers.

- Using the index finger, vibrate on the center of the tongue in a downward direction to flatten it. Stroke the tongue in a forward direction as index finger is withdrawn to decrease tongue retraction.

- Vibrate the cheek (see Figure 5.7) and gently move forward while grasping the cheek between the index finger (inside the mouth) and middle finger (along the cheek) to decrease hypertonicity and reduce upper lip retraction (Morris & Klein, 1987).

When using vibration, the following considerations should be taken into account:

- Ensure that vibration is not too intense, because this may result in an undesired increase in tone, rigidity, or extensor spasm (discontinue if vibration results in an increase in hypertonicity).

- Use vibration with caution if the individual has epilepsy.

- Individuals with hydrocephalus should not receive this treatment.

- Vibration inside the mouth is not appropriate if the individual has a tonic bite reflex.

MANIPULATION

Manipulation techniques such as tapping, stroking, and patting are applied directly to the muscles, using fingertips only. Firm, even pressure should be applied throughout the procedures. A quick stretch along the muscle fibers may be useful for stimulating hypotonic muscles. Manipulation procedures are useful not only for their direct effect on facilitating normal movement patterns but also for improving oral function through increased oral awareness and discrimination.

Manipulation Procedures

- Stroke face firmly in a downward direction.

- Using the index finger, vibrate on the center of the tongue in a downward direction to flatten it. Stroke the tongue in a forward direction as index finger is withdrawn to decrease tongue retraction.

- Vibrate the cheek (see Figure 5.7) and gently move fingers forward while grasping the cheek between the index finger (inside the mouth) and middle finger (along the cheek) to decrease hypertonicity and reduce upper lip retraction (Morris & Klein, 1987).

When using vibration, the following considerations should be taken into account:

- Ensure that vibration is not too intense, because this may result in an undesired increase in tone, rigidity, or extensor spasm (discontinue if vibration results in an increase in hypertonicity).

- Use with caution if the individual has epilepsy.

- Individuals with hydrocephalus should not receive this treatment.

- Vibration inside the mouth is not appropriate if the individual has a tonic bite reflex.

- Wipe the individual's face with a towel, maintaining constant, even pressure. This is particularly useful for individuals who are hypersensitive and have lip retraction due to increased tone (Morris & Klein, 1987).

- Flick the cheeks firmly but gently in an upward direction.

- Pull the bottom lip up flush against the upper lip.

- Pull the tongue (in a piece of gauze) and shake it gently before returning it to the mouth. If necessary, facilitate lip closure afterward.

- Tap under the chin in an upward direction to facilitate an increase in tone in a hypotonic tongue and to improve tongue stability.

- Tap the tongue, the cheeks, and around the mouth in a regular, rhythmic manner. This is particularly useful for individuals with a hypotonic face. Tap directly around the temporomandibular joint to increase jaw stability.

- Stroke the upper and lower gums, using firm, even pressure. Grade the pressure as necessary if the individual is hypersensitive.

- Stroke the tongue in a forward direction and the inside of the cheeks in a downward direction using firm, even pressure to decrease tone in hypertonic muscles.

- Make small circular movements around the mouth and under the chin. Do not press the larynx.
- Lift the larynx from below the thyroid cartilage to stimulate a reflex swallow. This procedure is useful to facilitate a swallow in individuals who do not have a spontaneous swallow.

Discontinue these techniques if stimulation results in hypertonicity in the oral–facial area or other parts of the body.

ORAL SENSORY–MOTOR EXERCISES

The following suggestions are exercises and activities that may be incorporated into an individual's program to improve oral–motor function, with the ultimate aim of improving saliva control. These exercises should immediately follow oral–facial facilitation techniques. The complexity of the oral exercise can be heightened by increasing the difficulty of the gross-motor activity once the fine-motor activity is achieved, for example, making faces in the mirror when sitting, when standing, when on one leg, and so forth.

Developing Lip Function

There is some evidence (Asher & Winquist, 1994; Fränkel & Fränkel, 1983; Moulding & Koroluk, 1991) that working toward a more competent lip seal may assist in controlling saliva and other fluids. Alteration of posture and jaw control and developing sensory–motor feedback already have been described. In addition, prostheses, such as an appliance in the vestibule to align the lips (oral or vestibular screen) or full intraoral appliances, such as ISMARs (Innsbrick Sensori Motor Activator and Regulator), can be used (see Chapter 8). Stavridi and Ahlgren (1992) suggested muscle responses to individualized oral screens increased the masseter and reduced the mentalis during swallowing. The lip pads increased the mentalis during lip seal but reduced the mentalis activity on swallowing. Lip pressure has been noted to change depending on the position of the head (Hellsing & L'Estrange, 1987). The increases in lip pressure in extension and decreases in flexion reinforce the importance of developing improved lip posture when the head is in a neutral position. Owman-Moll and Ingervall (1984) demonstrated that 10 minutes of practice twice a day improved lip strength.

 CASE STUDY

Alfonso was 13 years old and attended a mainstream school. He had some learning difficulties and a problem with saliva control. He really loved music and wanted to learn to play the trombone. The music teacher noticed how lax his lips were and tried hard to teach him. It took Alfonso 6 months to learn to play a few notes—he was very keen and kept on trying. After a while, his teacher noticed he no longer dribbled and his facial expression had improved.

Lip Exercises

- Make faces in the mirror, making various shapes with lips (e.g., smiling, pursing, kissing).

- Put lipstick or flavored lip gloss on the lips. Make a print on a tissue and examine the lip print (Marshalla, 1997).

- Hold a spatula or piece of paper between lips for an increasing length of time.

- Use a wide-diameter straw to suck up thickened fluids (e.g., pureed apple or tissue paper) and blow items such as paper and cotton wool (facilitation of lip closure may be necessary).

These exercises also require adequate velopharyngeal (i.e., soft palate against the pharyngeal wall) closure.

- Breathe like a fish—lips open and close. Start very slowly and increase the speed.

- Place foods such as jam on the top lip and encourage removal with the bottom lip.

- Incorporate the oral screen into practice. Start with a few minutes while reading a book or watching television and increase the length of time. The Exeter lip sensor also can be used.

- Thread a rubber band or string through a button and play a game in which the child holds the button between the lips while you pull lightly on the rubber band (Garliner, 1974).

Incorporate blowing games.

- Blow candles.

- Blow small cotton balls or little pieces of tissue across the table. This can be made into a "football" game in which you score goals.

- Using Ping-Pong balls and an egg carton, blow a Ping-Pong ball from one indentation to another.

- Blow bubbles.

- Musical instruments: Start with those instruments requiring little effort, for example, mouth organ, to one that requires more complex specificity, for example, trumpet. (Oetter et al., 1995).

Tongue Exercises

- Encourage food to be licked from specific sites using the tongue only. Place the food (e.g., jam or honey) at various sites inside the mouth and on and around the lips.

- Encourage the person to lick food from a plate or off the end of a spatula held in front of the mouth. (An ice cream stick or cone can be very motivating!)

- Encourage the person to lick envelopes, stickers, lollipops, and so on. (Facilitation of tongue movements may be necessary for some of these exercises. This can be done by moving the tongue with a craft stick or your finger.)

- Place small pieces of cracker in the pouch of each cheek.

- Use an electric toothbrush to massage the gums.

- Make up stories to motivate children about Mr. Tongue. For example,

> Mr. (or Ms.) tongue goes for a walk. He opens the door (open mouth), he walks out the door (poke out the tongue), he looks from right to left (move tongue from side to side), then he crosses the road (protrude tongue further), he walks up the hill (tongue up), and then down the hill (tongue down), he looks all around him (tongue circles lips), and then he goes home (tongue in and still), he has a drink (lap up some water), cleans his teeth (rub tongue over teeth), and then he goes to bed (finish with a swallow).

Developing Sensory Awareness

- Apply different textures to the face, such as shaving cream, fur, textured plastic or rubber items, rice, or soap suds. Introduce only one texture at a time. This can be developed into a game in which the child identifies the texture. Then increase the number of textures applied at any one time and have the child identify them.

- For children, encourage oral exploration and mouthing of toys or foods of various textures. Ensure that the toys are nontoxic and are not small enough to be inhaled.

DEVISING AN ORAL–FACIAL FACILITATION PROGRAM FOR YOUR CLIENT

When designing an oral–facial facilitation program for your client, it is important to consider the following: a trial of facilitation techniques; the frequency, length, and timing of the program; the training of the client, caregiver(s), and significant others implementing the program; and monitoring the effectiveness of the program. Do not try all four techniques at once. Choose one technique at a time and evaluate its effectiveness. A trial of three sessions should be adequate to determine its effectiveness.

Carefully grade the stimulation to increase tolerance, because some individuals may be sensitive to intense stimulation. You may present stimulation to other parts of the body as a preliminary introduction to the quality and intensity of the stimulus prior to presentation to the oral–facial area.

If, after a reasonable trial, the results are minimal or not significant, discontinue the trial and introduce another of the techniques. Once the trials have been completed, choose the technique that was most effective or a combination of effective techniques to implement as a part of the individual's daily routine.

IMPLEMENTATION OF THE PROGRAM

Once the program has been devised and implementation begins, it must be carefully monitored and regularly reviewed. The program should be implemented at least three times daily, and it initially should be introduced for short periods until there is an increase in tolerance to the stimulation. Take advantage of daily routines, such as mealtimes and teethbrushing times, to implement some of the techniques that have been outlined. Not only does this allow for treatment to take place in natural situations but also it facilitates the consistent implementation of the program at regular and routine intervals. Using the concepts of "facials" and "putting on makeup" are useful ways of implementing a more relaxed approach to sensory stimulation. For small children, bath time can be a relaxed time to play oral–motor games.

TRAINING

Caregivers and significant others should be trained in the implementation of the oral–facial facilitation program. They also should be trained to observe and record the effects of the program and provide appropriate reinforcement to the individual receiving treatment. Examples of written caregiver training materials can be found in Appendix A.

PROGRAM EVALUATION

It has been shown that oral–facial facilitation techniques are effective in reducing, but not always eliminating, drooling. These techniques serve to improve oral–motor function through intensive sensory stimulation. They also increase oral awareness and discrimination. When developing an oral–facial facilitation program, it is important to trial and evaluate the effectiveness of the techniques implemented and modify the program according to the responses and needs of the client.

EXAMPLES OF ORAL–FACIAL FACILITATION PROGRAMS

The following two programs are examples of how various oral–facial facilitation techniques can be used. The first program is adapted from a workshop presented by Margaret Rood in London, Ontario, Canada, in 1973.

Program 1

The following equipment is required: battery brush or medium-sized paintbrush, iced cotton balls or narrow ice molds, small hand towel or face cloth, 1-cm-wide stainless steel blade, and plastic straw or tubing about 3/4-mm wide.

1. Apply pressure and stretching around the mouth (see Figure 5.8). Avoid touching the lips.

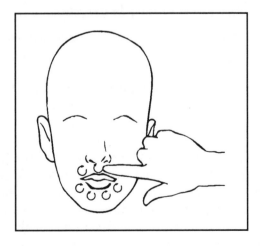

FIGURE 5.8. Pressure and stretching around the mouth.

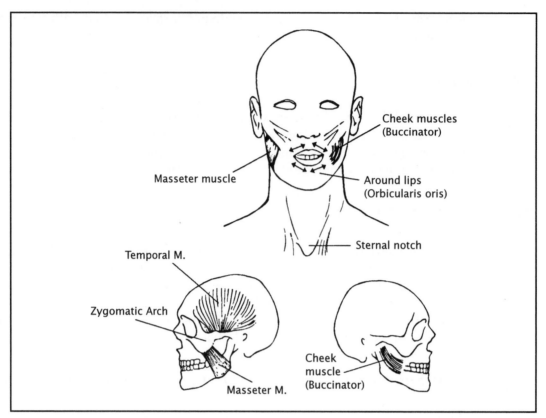

FIGURE 5.9. Brushing around the mouth and the cheek muscles.

2. Brush around the lips (orbicularis oris), along the cheeks (buccinators), and over the masseter (see Figure 5.9). Brush for a few seconds on each muscle group on each side of the face.

3. Thirty seconds later, apply ice with frozen treat. Mop dry after each swipe to stop the drips.

4. Repeat pressure and stretching around the mouth (orbicularis oris).

5. Three times, walk a stainless steel blade back along tongue (see Figure 5.10) to the beginning of the gag reflex. (Avoid eliciting the gag reflex.)

6. Slip the iced cotton swab from tip of tongue to the back along the central groove.

7. Swiftly stroke ice up across the sternal notch.

8. Have the client suck baby applesauce or soft ice cream up a straw or from the tip of a spoon several times.

Program 2

Castillo-Morales is an Argentinian man who developed a type of therapy that he terms oral–facial regulation therapy. Initially he worked with children with Down syndrome and has widened his treatment to include people with cerebral palsy or who have had strokes (Limbrock, Hoyer, & Scheying, 1990). The therapy is widely used in Scandinavia and Europe and incorporates physical therapy, oral–facial manual therapy, and palatal plates (Sjögreen, 2001). This program prepares the head and neck for further treatment

FIGURE 5.10. Walking a stainless steel blade on the tongue.

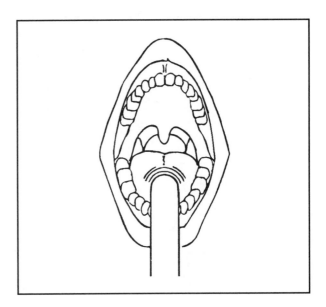

and may be best instituted at the start of each day. The best position for the individual is in supine. It is important to know and understand the anatomy of the head and neck. This program is best instituted with a trained Castillo-Morales therapist or physical therapist.

Motoric Calmness Exercise

1. With both hands under the scapula and the little finger on the inner side of the shoulder blade of the patient, make small vibration motions as hands are moved toward the shoulders.

2. Put hands on top of the patient's shoulders and press down with the fingers in time with the person's expiration, again using a small amount of vibration. This may be alternated by pressing on one shoulder and then another. (See Figure 5.11.)

3. Put hands on the front of the shoulder with hands pointing toward arms, press and vibrate with exhalation.

4. Take the head in hand, take all the weight and turn to the right, then the left. Ensure that the neck is kept long and straight. Be very gentle and careful. Do not tug or jerk.

5. Rotate the head gently left and then gently right.

6. Rotate the head slowly and carefully in a circle. The head must be fully supported.

7. With one hand on the occiput and one on the forehead, move hands toward each other and then away from each other.

8. Working from the top of the head (where the fontanel would have been), move the scalp in little circles with the thumbs.

9. With hands side by side on the frontalis, vibrate down toward the eyes (see Figure 5.12).

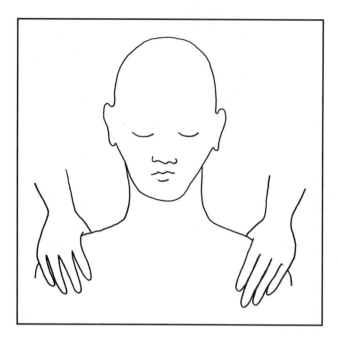

FIGURE 5.11. Position of hands on the shoulders.

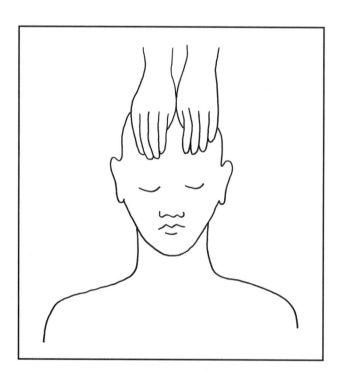

FIGURE 5.12. Vibrating down the forehead.

10. Work from the nose to outside of the eyes along the corrugator supercilii, giving extra stretch (flick when finished) at the eye end.

11. With the thumbs, work up the procerus (frown muscle).

12. Work around orbicularis oculi upper and lower, with an additional quick stretch by the eye.

13. Go down the levator labii superioris alaeque nasi with the thumbs and push out at the lip with a firm stretch.

14. Using the thumbs from midline to outside of mouth, follow orbicularis oris, upper and then lower.

15. Using the palm of the hands, move in and stretch on buccinator.

16. With cupped hands, use the tips of fingers back and forth to move orbicularis oris.

17. With the flat of hand, push down and pull up on the side of the chin.

18. With the fingertips, make rotating movements on the mentalis.

19. Use the fingertips on the floor of the mouth under the chin, followed with vibration of the whole hand. Only use vibration if the jaw is protruded.

20. Put the head back, then forward, and then sideways. Hold firmly. To obtain lateral movements, put two fingers on the side of the mandible and turn the head to the midline with flexion while the person resists.

REFERENCES

Asher, R. S., & Winquist, H. (1994). Appliance therapy for chronic drooling in a patient with mental retardation. *Special Care in Dentistry, 14*(1), 30–32.

Ayers, J. (1979). *Sensory integration and the child.* Los Angeles: Western Psychological Services.

Carlstedt, K., Dahllöf, G., Nilsson, B., & Modeer, T. (1996). Effect of palatal plate therapy in children with Down syndrome. *Acta Odontology Scandinavia, 54*, 122–125.

Domaracki, L. S., & Sisson, L. A. (1990). Decreasing drooling with oral motor stimulation in children with multiple disabilities. *American Journal of Occupational Therapy, 44*(8), 680–684.

Draper, M. (1968, May). Aids to improving vocalization. *New Zealand Journal of Physiotherapy,* 11–17.

Falk, M. L., Wells, M., & Toth, S. (1976). A subcortical approach to swallow pattern therapy. *American Journal of Orthodontics, 70*(4), 419–427.

Fischer-Brandies, H., Avalle, C., & Limbrock, G. J. (1987). Therapy of orofacial dysfunctions in cerebral palsy according to Castillo-Morales: First results of a new treatment concept. *European Orthodontic Society, 9*, 139–143.

Fränkel, R., & Fränkel, C. (1983). A functional approach to treatment of skeletal open bite. *American Journal of Orthodontics, 84*(1), 54–68.

Gallender, D. (1979). *Eating handicaps: Illustrated techniques for feeding disorders.* Springfield, IL: Thomas.

Garliner, D. (1974). *Myofunctional therapy in dental practice.* Coral Gables, FL: Institute for Myofunctional Therapy.

Gisel, E. G. (1996). Effect of oral sensorimotor treatment on measures of growth and efficiency of eating in the moderately eating-impaired child with cerebral palsy. *Dysphagia, 11*(1), 48–58.

Gisel, E. G., Applegate-Ferrante, T., Benson, J., & Bosma, J. (1996). Oral–motor skills following sensori motor therapy in two groups of moderately dysphagic children with cerebral palsy: Aspiration vs non aspiration. *Dysphagia, 11*(1), 59–71.

Grant, L. (1982). The use of a manual vibrator in the speech therapy program of four school-age mentally retarded children. *Journal of Communication Disorders, 15*(5), 375–383.

Haberfellner, H., Schwartz, S. T., & Gisel, E. G. (2001). Feeding skills and growth after one year on intra-oral appliance therapy in moderately dysphagic children with cerebral palsy. *Dysphagia, 16*(2), 83–96.

Hamer, J. L. (1972, August). Ice therapy—A review. *New Zealand Journal of Physiotherapy,* 37–38.

Hellsing, E., & L'Estrange, P. (1987). Changes in lip pressure following extension and flexion of the head and at changed mode of breathing. *American Journal of Orthodontic Dentofacial and Orthopaedics, 91*, 286–294.

Langley, J. (1987). *Working with swallowing disorders.* Bicester, Oxon, England: Winslow Press.

Limbrock, G. J., Fischer-Brandies, H., & Avalle, C. (1991). Castillo-Morales' orofacial therapy: Treatment of 67 children with Down syndrome. *Developmental Medicine and Child Neurology, 33*(4), 296–303.

Limbrock, G. J., Hoyer, H., & Scheying, H. (1990, November/December). Drooling, chewing and swallowing dysfunctions in children with cerebral palsy: Treatment according to Castillo-Morales. *Journal of Dentistry for Children,* 445–451.

Logeman, J. A. (1983). Anatomy and physiology of normal deglutition. In J. A. Logeman, (Ed.), *Evaluation and treatment of swallowing disorders.* San Diego, CA: College Hill Press.

Loiselle, C. (1979). Rood-based program for decreasing pre-feeding behaviours. *Canadian Journal of Occupational Therapy, 46*(3), 93–98.

Marshalla, P. (1997). *Drooling. Guidelines and activities.* Temecula, CA: Speech Dynamics.

Morris, S. E., & Klein, M. D. (1987). *Pre-feeding skills.* Tucson, AZ: Communication Skills Builder.

Morton, R. E., Bonas, R., Fourie, B., & Minford, J. (1993). Videofluoroscopy in the assessment of feeding disorders of children with neurological problems. *Developmental Medicine and Child Neurology, 35*(5), 388–395.

Moulding, M. B., & Koroluk, L. D. (1991). An intraoral prosthesis to control drooling in a patient with amytrophic lateral sclerosis. *Special Care in Dentistry, 11*(5), 200–202.

Oetter, P., Richter, E. W., & Frick, S. M. (1995). *M.O.R.E. Integrating the mouth with sensory and postural functions* (2nd. ed.). Hugo, MN: PDP.

Owman-Moll, P., & Ingervall, B. (1984). Effect of oral screen treatment on dentition, lip morphology and function in children with incompetent lips. *American Journal of Orthodontics, 85*(1), 37–46.

Rantala, S. (2001). Foniatrician in the orofacial treatment team. In M. Sillanpä (Ed.), *Practices on orofacial therapy* (pp. 11–15). Helsinki, Finland: Finnish Association of Orofacial Therapy.

Rood, M. S. (1954). Neurophysiological reactions as a basis for physical therapy. *Physical Therapy Review, 34,* 444–449.

Russell, B. (2001). Perioral and oral stimulation in dysphagia—The Vangede concept and stimulation according to Russell. In M. Sillanpä (Ed.), *Practices on orofacial therapy* (pp. 39–40). Helsinki, Finland: Finnish Association of Orofacial Therapy.

Sjögreen, L. (2001). Speech therapist in the orofacial treatment team. In M. Sillanpä (Ed.), *Practices on orofacial therapy* (pp. 11–15). Helsinki, Finland: Finnish Association of Orofacial Therapy.

Stavridi, R., & Ahlgren, J. (1992). Muscle response to the oral screen activator. An EMG study of the masseter, buccinator and mentalis muscles. *European Journal of Orthodontics, 14,* 339–349.

CHAPTER

Behavioral Approaches to Saliva Control

Learning Outcomes

- *Define a behavioral learning program*

- *Describe three factors that may affect the efficacy of a behavioral program*

- *Outline the component phases of a behavioral program*

- *Name four behaviors that may be targeted in a saliva-control behavioral learning program*

- *List a primary, secondary, and generalized reinforcer*

- *Describe one device that may be used in a behavioral program*

LEARNING ABOUT SALIVA CONTROL

Candidates for behavioral therapy may be identified by answers to Questions 3 to 5, 10, and 16 on the Saliva Control Assessment form (see Appendix A).

Behavioral therapy, or the learning of a new behavior, can be the first step in therapy for saliva control, or it can be used in conjunction with another therapy (e.g., medication). Many people choose behavioral intervention over other interventions because they perceive it to be noninvasive and unlikely to have side effects. This is not necessarily true. Successful behavioral therapy requires commitment from all parties involved, requires consistent and persistent effort, and may be unpleasant for the client or other people involved. Side effects also can occur, for example, a sore chin may be an unwanted side effect of a behavioral program for chin wiping. The level of success achieved will depend on a variety of factors, and it may seem unworthy of the efforts made. However, even partial success may be enough to affect the perception of the severity of the problem. For example, increasing lip closure and swallowing behavior may be achieved in a program but may be maintained by the client for short periods of time only. Muscle fatigue and inability to maintain concentration may mean the client can stay dry for only

2 hours at a time. However, when the client goes to the movies with his or her friends every Saturday, this level of success is enough to make a perceptible difference to his or her life.

Many successful behavioral programs have been reported. Behaviors that have been targeted and that have shown varying degrees of success are chin wiping (Drabmen, Cordua y Cruz, Ross, & Lynd, 1979; Dunn, Cunningham, & Backman, 1987; Lancioni, Brouwer, & Coninx, 1994; Lancioni, Connix, Manders, & Driessen, 1989), self-awareness of the need to swallow (Dunn et al. 1987), improved swallowing and oral–motor functioning (Helfrich-Miller, Rector, & Straka, 1986; Koheil, Sochaniwskyj, Bablich, Kenny, & Milner, 1987), increased frequency of swallow (Koheil et al., 1987), and improved lip closure (Callinan, Snelleman, & Vincent, 1986; Huskie et al., 1981). Small subject numbers and "lack of scientific rigor" (S. R. Harris & Purdy, 1987) have made it difficult to draw any serious conclusions about the efficacy of one treatment method over another.

Another variable in the research has been the prompts used, which can include auditory cues such as tones or buzzers (Koheil et al., 1987; Lancioni et al., 1994), physical cues such as chin cups or lip electrodes to promote jaw and lip closure (Callinan et al., 1986; M. M. Harris & Dignam, 1980), and self-monitoring (Dunn et al., 1987). Reinforcements have ranged from tokens, music, social praise, and verbal self-rewards to criticism, scolding, and overcorrection (Drabman et al., 1979; Dunn et al., 1987). All of these approaches have reported degrees of success over the short term.

WHO WILL BENEFIT?

A behavioral program implies the learning and integration of a new skill, and the literature on saliva control has suggested that success with a behavioral program relies on certain basic cognitive ability. The published research has shown varying degrees of success with a wide variety of individuals, methods, and intensities of treatment. The subjects of the research have varied enormously, from those with no cognitive impairment but with mild physical difficulties to those with profound impairments of both cognitive function and physical abilities (Helfrich-Miller et al., 1986), and they have still shown success.

Personality also may affect the success of a behavioral program with traits such as compliance and sensitivity to social approval being possible predictors of success (Lancioni et al., 1994). Other predictors of success for behavioral intervention have been identified as reduced oral–motor involvement, some mobility, and age—that is, old enough to understand what is requested (Thomas-Stonell & Greenberg, 1988). Behavioral therapy can be seen in the context of a continuum of learning theory (see Figure 6.1). This continuum has two sides.

The right-hand side of the continuum is the learning and integration of a new behavior because it has positive and perceivable consequences for the learner. These conse-

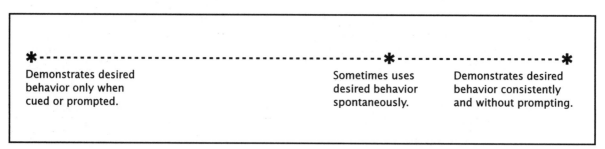

FIGURE 6.1. Continuum of learning theory.

quences result in consistent use of the new behavior because the learner is internally motivated to use the new learning.

The left-hand side of the continuum is when learning theory has been applied, but individuals may not yet have perceived any reason for learning a new behavior. They may have learned the behavior or skill and used it in some situations or with some cuing, but they have not learned that the behavior has positive consequences for them and they do not choose to use their skill spontaneously or cannot maintain it consistently. This pure form of learning theory is difficult to apply to saliva control issues. Many people might argue that people whose behaviors meet the criteria of the left side of the continuum have been unsuccessful in their behavioral program. Rather, this may be seen as success in teaching a compensatory behavior, but a further program may be required to motivate the person to internalize the skills. Some researchers claim that success has been achieved with saliva control problems over the long term even when cuing is still required to achieve optimum control (Lancioni et al., 1994).

For some people, the connection between a behavior and a desirable consequence cannot be internalized, because they do not have a full understanding of cause and effect or they may not have the physical skills to maintain the behavior over time. The indicators for success with a program lie in tailoring the treatment to suit the skills, motivation, interests, and cognitive level of each individual (Thomas-Stonell & Greenberg, 1988). Ensuring that goals are clear and that people involved in the implementation understand their roles and are committed to the goals also are vital to success.

WHAT IS A BEHAVIORAL LEARNING PROGRAM?

A behavioral learning program is designed to increase, decrease, or stop the occurrence of a specific behavior. For example, a program aimed at losing weight may include learning to decrease eating behaviors or to increase exercise behavior. Similarly, a saliva control program may aim to increase swallowing behavior, decrease open-mouth behavior, or stop "hands-in-mouth" behavior. Behavioral learning programs consist of specific phases, no matter what behavior is being targeted for new learning. These phases include the following:

- selecting the behavior to be changed;

- measuring the behavior;

- planning and preparing, which includes choosing a key worker, defining goals, planning for evaluation within the program, choosing the appropriate reinforcements, choosing the schedule of timing, and gathering any necessary equipment;

- administering the program, which includes shaping, prompting, and fading the prompts; and

- generalizing and maintaining the behaviors.

WHICH BEHAVIOR DO I WANT TO CHANGE?

Specific behaviors that have been targeted in saliva control programs include:

- learning to maintain better head posture (Thomas-Stonell & Greenberg, 1988);

- learning lip closure and jaw stability (S. R. Harris & Purdy, 1987; Helfrich-Miller et al., 1986; Thomas-Stonell & Greenberg, 1988);

- learning more effective swallowing, including chewing, eating, and intraoral pressure (Dunn et al., 1987; Koheil et al., 1987; Thorbecke & Jackson, 1982); and

- learning effective chin wiping or mouth wiping (Drabmen et al., 1979; Lancioni et al., 1989, 1994; Rapp, 1980).

There may be a variety of behaviors contributing to the problem, so it is important to describe the behaviors carefully and decide which one is contributing most to the problem.

 CASE STUDY

Carmella is a young woman with a severe intellectual disability. She has poor oral muscle tone, which results in poor lip closure and inefficient swallowing. She also has a habit of putting her fisted right hand into her mouth as part of her self-engagement behavior. In several situations, Carmella's loss of saliva was mild when her hands were occupied and moderate to severe when she had her hand in her mouth. It was decided that a behavioral program to reduce her "hands-in-mouth" behavior was the most appropriate.

The potential for changing the behavior also may be a deciding factor. In this case, all parties agreed that keeping Carmella busy was something that could be done fairly easily, and her hand-in-mouth behavior would then be reduced.

MEASURING THE BEHAVIOR

To determine if the learning program has been effective, it is important to measure and describe the behavior so there is a baseline against which to measure change. You may choose to measure the behavior you wish to teach (e.g., lips together) or the contingent behavior that is the presenting problem (i.e., loss of saliva). If you choose to measure loss of saliva as the presenting problem, then you must be confident that the skill you choose to teach will help solve the problem. If you have taught the skill and there is no change in levels of saliva loss, then you may have chosen a behavior that was irrelevant to loss of saliva. Also, the person must be physically capable of performing the behavior. Will a child with low muscle tone in his or her lips ever be able to learn "lips together" as a behavior? Or would a compensatory mouth-wiping program be more effective? You may need to teach more than one new skill to alleviate the problem (e.g., better head posture, more frequent swallowing), so measuring the saliva loss will give you the most information about which behavior is contributing most to the problem. (More information about measuring and describing techniques is provided in Chapter 3.)

PLANNING AND PREPARATION

The planning stage may involve a team of people who know the person well (e.g., parents, teachers, friends, neighbors, siblings, coworkers, staff, work supervisors). This team helps ensure that the most realistic assessment of the person's skills, motivation, interests, and cognitive level are taken into account in the planning.

DECIDING ON A KEY WORKER

Behavioral programs require consistency and persistence. There must be at least one person who can spend time with the client on a daily basis and who is prepared to be persistent in the administration of the program. This person needs to be integrally involved in the planning and setting of goals so that there is a personal investment in the outcomes. The key person may require training and access to other members of the planning team for advice, problem solving, and ongoing support. The key person may be a teacher, teacher's aide, parent, coworker, supervisor, or any person who understands the program goals and who is able to spend time administering the program. The key person may need training in

- observing behaviors and responses to provide appropriate feedback;

- differentiating responses so that the "best" skill or behavior can be shaped and rewarded;

- rewarding and responding at the appropriate time and with the "right amount" of reward; or

- measuring and describing. The key worker must not rely totally on human judgment or unstructured impressions. Actual frequency of behaviors often is misjudged depending on the mood or the memory of the person reporting if complete, objective records are not maintained.

DEFINING GOALS

In planning goals, not only does the skill to be learned need to be identified but also the situations in which the skill or behavior should or should not occur need to be identified. The goals must be objective and describe observable characteristics of the skill or behavior. For example, Eamon will learn to close his lips together and swallow (with lips together) when requested. The goals need to be clear and unambiguous. They also need to be complete. Delineate boundary conditions. For example, Miho will learn to lift her head to an upright and midline position when staff say, "Head up, Miho," only when Miho is seated in her postured work chair. It is important that specific, observable skills or behaviors, rather than the global idea of "drooling," become the target of the learning program. A specified behavior is much easier to deal with than general impressions.

EVALUATION

In planning the program, it is important to have ongoing evaluation built in as part of the procedure. This evaluation usually involves measuring changes in the frequency of target skills or changes in the contingent behaviors. The information obtained in these measurements may indicate that goals need to be altered. For example, if teaching the reduction of hands-in-mouth behavior as a new skill was having no impact on the level of saliva loss, then either the relevance of the skill or the effectiveness of the teaching would need to be revised.

MOTIVATION TO LEARN, OR "DIFFERENT STROKES FOR DIFFERENT FOLKS"

Appropriate and motivating consequences or reinforcers can make or break a program. This is one reason why it is important to know the person well in order to assess what in particular will be a motivating reinforcer.

➡ Examples

- Filipo loves physical contact and interacting with people. Verbal praise and a pat on the back are appropriate reinforcers for Filipo.

- Julia does not like being touched and does not enjoy being with people. Filipo's reinforcers would not be rewarding for Julia.

Types of Consequences or Reinforcers

There are two main types of reinforcement: positive and negative.

A positive reinforcer is an event presented after a behavior has been performed that increases the frequency of that particular behavior.

➡ Examples

- Julio lifts up his head, and his mother responds by turning on the television. Julio lifts up his head more often.

- Sally closes her lips and swallows, and her workshop supervisor responds by smiling at her and saying how pretty Sally looks today. Sally's lip closure increases and she swallows more often.

A negative reinforcer is an event that is removed after a behavior has been performed that decreases the frequency of that behavior.

➡ Examples

- Spiros wears a lip sensor that emits an unpleasant buzz if his lips are parted. When he closes his lips, the noise stops. Spiros does not like the noise, so he keeps his lips together.

- Kieran is embarrassed by his mother's constant comments on his saliva and her patronizing wiping of his chin. Kieran begins swallowing more when he is with his mother and generally stays dry, and his mother's comments and wipings cease.

For the purposes of saliva control programs, positive reinforcers are easier to plan for and administer than negative reinforcers, but occasionally a negative reinforcer may be appropriate.

WHICH REINFORCER IS MOST POWERFULLY MOTIVATING?

Reinforcers can be further categorized into primary, secondary (or conditioned), and generalized conditioned reinforcers.

Primary reinforcers involve basic physical needs and sensations, for example, food or drink (positive reinforcers) or shock or loud noise (negative reinforcers). *Secondary reinforcers* have to be conditioned (e.g., praise, money). *Generalized conditioned reinforcers* have a variety of reinforcing events contributing to their value and are generally the most useful, if they are motivating to the client (e.g., attention). James (1992) noted that the pairing of social reinforcement with a reinforcer contingent on the desired behavior (activated music when the head is up) creates a marked impact on retention of the skill.

⮞ Examples

- Tokens, chips, or money can buy a variety of rewarding events such as TV, snacks, or outings.

- Attention or approval may bring associated reinforcers, for example, physical contact, praise, or smiles.

The best reinforcement is the motivation that comes from achieving the skill and all the positive responses that occur with new learning (e.g., praise, inclusion, and independence). Reinforcers also can consist of food or consumables, social high-probability behaviors, feedback, and tokens. Table 6.1 lists examples of each of these reinforcers and lists pros and cons of the different types of reinforcers.

DEVICES AND EQUIPMENT

Electronic devices and equipment may be used to help in behavioral programs. Devices generally have been used as prompts or reinforcers and occasionally in evaluation relating to specific saliva control behaviors.

The Accularm (Koheil et al., 1987) is a device that emits a sound at regular intervals to remind the user to perform whatever behavior is being targeted to help the control of saliva, for example, keeping the lips together, lifting up the head, swallowing, sucking back the saliva then swallowing, removing fingers from the mouth, and so forth. The battery-operated device emits a tone through an earpiece at intervals, ranging between 5 and 120 seconds. These intervals can be changed to provide various schedules of prompt depending on what phase of the behavioral program is occurring (more beeps for prompting, fewer in the fading and generalization phases). This tone is a cue or prompt, and when the prompt is removed there may be generalization or no generalization of the desired behavior. Research has shown this device to be effective for a group of subjects who were selectively chosen for their cognitive, physical, and oral abilities, because they were able to comply with directions and change their swallowing behavior (Thomas-Stonell & Greenberg, 1988). This device also can double as an evaluation device, because the key worker can wear it and observe the client, noting if targeted behaviors are present at each beep over a specific period of time. This can be repeated later in the program to see if there are any measurable, numerically quantifiable changes in the targeted behaviors

TABLE 6.1
List of Reinforcers

Type of Reinforcer	Samples and Ideas	Pro	Con
Food consumable	Lollipops, cookies, gum, drinks	• Paired with social so that the secondary reinforcers are built to a strong level	• Dependent on deprivation state • Interrupts ongoing behavior • Difficult to give immediately • Ethical issues of depriving of food, and so on • May increase drooling
Social	Verbal praise, attention, physical contact (touching, pats, hand-holding), facial expression (smile, eye contact, nods, wink)	• Easily given • Portable • Naturally occurring • Generalized reinforcer	• May not be naturally reinforcing
High probability	Playing with friends, watching TV, listening to music, playing a game		• Ethical issues of depriving a person who may already have limited control over life • Need a good cognitive understanding
Feedback	Can be paired with food, social, and so on, or can be given by itself • Auditory (verbal, sound) • Visual (scales, chat)	• Can be paired with a variety of other reinforcers • Can be naturally occurring and therefore maintain behavior	
Tokens	Money, chips, stamps, buttons	• Very potent • Generalized reinforcer • Can be traded for a variety of motivating activities • Can be used to set up a delay in delivery of reward	• Hard to fade • Not naturally occurring • Not immediately rewarding, need to have ability to abstract to future event. Delay may not be understood.

rather than relying on observational, descriptive data only. The Accularm is available from the Bloorview MacMillan center, Electronics Program, Rehabilitation Engineering Department, Canada.

The Exeter lip sensor is a device used in saliva control programs for people who require lip closure as their target behavior (Callinan et al., 1986; Huskie et al., 1981; see Figure 6.2). The device is a lip electrode that hooks onto the lower lip and emits a buzzing sound (negative reinforcer that prompts to close lips) each time the person parts the lips and the lip seal and electrode connection is broken. An alternative form of the

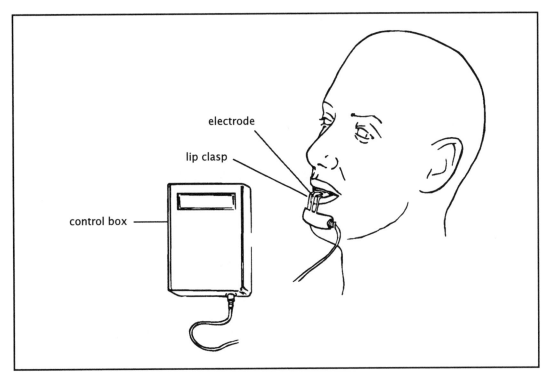

FIGURE 6.2. Exeter lip sensor.

device also can be connected to a small radio or tape player to provide positive reinforcement (e.g., favorite music or radio station instead of the buzzer) when the lips remain closed. The individual's use of the sensor determines the schedule of the program because the positive reinforcement is continuous and the negative reinforcement or prompt buzz sound occurs each time the lips part. Research results are inconclusive, claiming that people with good cognitive skills and no physical impairment may do well with the device, whereas those with either physical impairment or cognitive impairment will have a lesser result. Huskie et al. (1981) and Callinan et al. (1986) demonstrated that a lip seal could be achieved with two cognitively able children but that only one child was able to maintain the behavior.

SCHEDULES—IT'S ALL IN THE TIMING

Once the goals have been set and the reinforcement type decided, a schedule of reinforcement must be planned. There are many ways of administering the reinforcements, and the schedule may need to change during different parts of the program.

Continuous reinforcement consists of a simple schedule in which reinforcement is given each time the desired behavior occurs. While a behavior is developing, continuous reinforcement helps the person to perform the behavior at a higher rate. (Behaviors that have been continuously reinforced also deteriorate quickly when the reinforcement is removed.)

Intermittent reinforcement is when the reinforcement is delivered only after the desired behavior has occurred several times. On an intermittent schedule, occurrence of the behavior continues for a longer period of time even after the reinforcement has ceased. Intermittent reinforcement has the benefits of efficiently using reinforcers, being less time-consuming than administered continuous reinforcements, and having little risk of boredom or satiation with the reinforcer.

Ratio schedule and *interval schedule* are examples of intermittent reinforcement. A ratio schedule consists of giving reinforcement only after the desired behavior has occurred a specified number of times. For example, Maarit receives one star on her chart for every five times she closes her lips and swallows. An interval schedule is dependent upon the amount of time that passes before the reinforcement is given. Dina, for example, is given a token every 10 minutes if she sits up straight when her work supervisor looks over to check.

Interval schedules are easier to administer, but the individual's performance is usually higher under ratio schedules. Interval and ratio schedules may be fixed or variable. Variable ratio schedules are not easily extinguished and occur in real-life situations such as using slot machines or going fishing. Because there is no way of knowing when the reward is going to happen, the behavior continues at a high level (e.g., continuing to put money in the slot machine and waiting for a win, continuing to throw the fishing line in and waiting for a bite).

Generally, the best way to schedule reinforcement for a saliva control program is to start with a continuous (1:1) schedule until the desired behavior has been well established, then change to a ratio or interval schedule, and make the reinforcement more intermittent.

SHAPING, PROMPTING, AND FADING

Not all people are going to be highly motivated to learn new behavior. Many people may learn the behavior during the program, but if they do not understand the benefits that the behavior provides, the behavior may not continue.

When providing a program, it is important to define how much assistance the client will be given to learn the behavior. This assistance may take the form of shaping a desired behavior, prompting the behavior to occur, and then fading out the prompts. If motivation to learn the behavior and use the behavior is not evident at any stage, then fading out the prompts may not be a viable phase of the program.

Shaping

Shaping is the reinforcement of a behavior that approximates the behavior to be learned. For example, if someone is learning to swallow more regularly, then reinforcing "lips together" in preparation for swallowing is a shaping procedure. Even if the person does not follow the lip closure with a swallow, an attempt is being made and must be reinforced as a precursor to the desired behavior. Reinforcement of approximations gradually ceases and the person is fully reinforced only for swallowing.

Prompting

Prompting involves various ways of reminding the person to use the new skill or behavior. Prompts range from fully physically assisting the person to perform the skill to a conditioned reminder that is unrelated to the skill (e.g., swallowing when hearing a beep).

It is important to plan the sequence of prompts carefully so that the person can gradually become more independent in the learned skill use and not be reliant on continuous one-on-one prompting. For instance, if a person is learning a new head posture to control saliva, it is important that the prompts be reduced from, perhaps, full physical manipulation to attain correct head posture to a partial physical prompt, for instance, a gentle hand tap on the neck, then to a verbal or visual prompt of "head up." In reducing the strength of prompts, it is vital to ensure that success has been achieved at one level before moving to a lesser prompt.

When planning a program, keep in mind that a fine line exists between giving too many prompts, so that the person becomes reliant on prompting to initiate the skill, and not enough prompts, so that the behavior is used too infrequently to become integrated as a new skill. Several research articles (James, 1992; Koheil et al., 1987) recommend an adequate number of training sessions or "training to criteria" to enhance the chances of generalization and maintenance of the behavior.

Fading

Fading is the process in which prompts gradually become fewer as the person internalizes use of the new behavior. With successful learning, fading of prompts should eventually become complete. Fading needs to be gradual and prompts should be minimal or have ceased by the end of training.

GENERALIZATION AND MAINTENANCE

Generalization

Generalization of a skill may be a necessary phase in a behavioral learning program for saliva control. If a skill has been learned and practiced in one setting, it may or may not be used automatically in a different setting. For instance, someone may learn to stay dry in a social setting (e.g., out shopping with friends) but may not transfer this skill to daily activities at their day placement. A specific part of the program (or of a transfer program) may be designed to help generalize the use of a new skill in a variety of settings. Generalization may need to occur across places, times, or with various people. Generalization may not occur when cues or prompts are faded. Lancioni et al. (1994) discusses device-assisted success in which cues or prompts keep the success level high and the need to pair cues with social reinforcement to promote generalization of the behavior when specific cues are faded.

Maintenance

After administering a teaching program to a client, he or she has learned a new skill, the prompts have been faded, and the client is dry. Two weeks later, the client has a wet chin. What went wrong? Maybe the new skill had not really been internalized, or maybe the reinforcers were not occurring regularly enough in the natural environment. Perhaps there may be other factors in the environment that have upset the new learning so that it is not maintained. For example, a client who had achieved optimum swallow rate to stay dry is learning a new task in his or her work, and the concentration required has fatigued the client so that he or she cannot maintain the swallow rate.

Follow-up and maintenance programs need to be planned if long-term success is expected. Everyone needs support and encouragement to maintain change. Maintenance may be as simple as regular meetings and pep talks to reinforce new learning. Maintenance can occur in a self-help group to discuss problem times and to encourage people to maintain skill levels. Follow-up programs may be offered periodically to remind people of their skills. Maintenance of skills will be vastly different from person to person, so opportunities to revise and maintain must remain flexible. It may be wise to assign one person to monitor maintenance of the skills and report back if further intervention is required.

EXAMPLES OF BEHAVIORAL PROGRAMS

Behavior Program 1: Learning a New Head Posture

Client

William is a 35-year-old man with cerebral palsy who works in a supported employment setting. He has requested input from the speech–language pathologist, because he is distressed by the fact that he dribbles on finished paperwork.

Persons Responsible

William, his supervisor, and a speech–language pathologist are the persons responsible.

Behavior To Be Learned

The behavior William wants to learn is to keep his head upright and in the midline to reduce saliva loss.

Goal

The goal is for William to keep his head upright and in the midline when he is seated at his workbench, which is angled so that his work is at eye level. William agreed that this was a useful goal.

Measurement and Evaluation Schedule

- Week 1: The supervisor gives William new work or removes work he has completed approximately every 10 minutes. The supervisor is to check head posture and praise correct posture or remind William and physically assist posture if it is not correct. Drooling is measured once a week.

- Week 2: The supervisor picks up William's work every 20 minutes and charts the progress. William and his supervisor review each day's chart, and William graphs his own progress.

- Week 3: Every 30 minutes the supervisor charts progress. William continues daily review and charting.

Reinforcement

- May need to physically assist William to lift up his chin

- Prompt—touching William on his head to prompt head up

- Cue—When William looks at his direct supervisor, supervisor lifts up his own head

- Praise, smiles, and self-monitoring of daily results

- Monetary bonus at end of week for needing less than 20% percent reminders to maintain head posture

Generalization

The speech–language pathologist monitors William's head posture at lunchtime in the cafeteria in Week 4 of the program. In week 6, William's head posture is monitored at a football game. William is to self-monitor and report back to the speech–language pathologist on a situation of his choice.

Maintenance

Have a random week of charting and monitoring. William continues to receive a wage bonus if he maintains head posture.

Behavior Program 2: Learning To Swallow More Frequently

Client

José is a 4-year-old boy with low oral tone who swallows infrequently. His mother is worried he will still be drooling when he goes to school next year.

Persons Responsible

José's mother and a speech–language pathologist are the persons responsible.

Behavior To Be Learned

The behavior José wants to learn is to swallow more frequently in order to reduce saliva loss.

Goal

The goal is for José to swallow once every 2 minutes when he is sitting quietly, watching TV.

Measurement and Evaluation Schedule

José's saliva control is to be rated five times over 2 weeks before the program begins. José's saliva control is to be measured twice a week during the duration of the program and twice a week for 1 month after the program has ended. The program will last for 1 hour per day over 3 weeks. The total measurement and evaluation time is 9 weeks.

Shape, Prompt, and Fade

Shape. Before the program begins, José will spend three 20-minute sessions with the speech–language pathologist, learning how to swallow on request every 2 minutes. This can be done with a simple dice game in which José has to swallow when he hears the buzzer or speech–language pathologist's voice. Failure to swallow means José forfeits a turn. When José can swallow on request 10 times in 20 minutes, the program can begin.

Prompt. When José sits down to watch TV, his mother puts on a 1-hour audio-cassette that has the speech–language pathologist's voice instructing José to swallow and a beep accompanying the voice every 2 minutes. José's mother will monitor his swallow-ing in Week 1 at hours 1, 3, and 5 to shape his swallowing. In Week 2, she will monitor a random 30 minutes of hours 6, 8, and 10. In Week 3, José's mother will monitor a ran-dom 20 minutes of hours 12, 14, and 15.

Fade. When José is swallowing consistently 90% of the time in response to the tape, José will practice swallowing to a beep without the verbal reminder. During Week 3, the tape will be played for only 30 minutes of the hour that José is watching TV.

Reinforcement

José will receive a new toy car at the end of every week if he has achieved 90% swallow-ing during the time he was being monitored. José's mother will give him lots of praise for his swallowing and will make a chart using colored stickers to show him how many swallows he does each day.

Generalization

José can wear an ear plug attached to a beeper that is set to beep every 2 minutes. José may wear the ear plug for 30 minutes a day during different situations. After he has completed his program, the beep will act as a conditioned cue for him to swallow.

Maintenance

José's mother will secretly observe José's swallowing once a week for 15 minutes in a variety of situations. If José is swallowing fewer than once every 3 minutes, she may introduce the beeper each day for a week while he is watching TV.

A caregiver training material titled Helping Your Child Toward a Dry Chin can be found in Appendix B.

REFERENCES

Callinan, F., Snelleman, J., & Vincent, J. (1986). Clinical application of the lip sensor. *Australian Journal of Human Communication Disorders, 14*(2), 87–93.

Drabmen, R., Cordua y Cruz, G., Ross, J., Lynd, S. (1979). Suppression of chronic drooling in mentally retarded children and adolescents: Effectiveness of a behavioural treatment package. *Behaviour Therapy, 10*, 46–56.

Dunn, K. W., Cunningham, C. E., & Backman, J. E. (1987). Self-control and reinforcement in the management of a cerebral-palsied adolescent's drooling. *Developmental Medicine and Child Neurology, 29*(3), 305–310.

Harris, M. M., & Dignam, P. F. (1980). A non-surgical method of reducing drooling in cerebral-palsied children. *Developmental Medicine and Child Neurology, 22*(3), 293–299.

Harris, S. R., & Purdy, A. H. (1987). Drooling and its management in cerebral palsy. *Developmental Medicine and Child Neurology, 29*(6), 807–811.

Helfrich-Miller, K. R., Rector, K. L., & Straka, J. A. (1986). Dysphagia: Its treatment in the profoundly retarded patient with cerebral palsy. *Archives of Physical Medicine and Rehabilitation, 67*, 520–525.

Huskie, C. F., Ellis, R. E., Flack, F. C., Coutts, S. E., Dangerfield, A. W., & Selley, W. G. (1981, November). The Exeter lip sensor in clinical use—Work in progress—Part 1. *Bulletin of College of Speech and Language Therapists, 335*, 1–6.

James, R. (1992). Biofeedback treatment for cerebral palsy in children and adolescents: A review. *Paediatric Exercise Science, 4*, 198–212.

Koheil, R., Sochaniwskyj, A. E., Bablich, K., Kenny, D. J., & Milner, M. (1987). Biofeedback techniques and behaviour modification in the conservative remediation of drooling by children with cerebral palsy. *Developmental Medicine and Child Neurology, 29*(1), 19–26.

Lancioni, G. E., Brouwer, J. A., & Coninx, F. (1994). Automatic cueing to reduce drooling: A long-term follow up with two mentally handicapped persons. *Journal of Behavior Therapy and Experimental Psychiatry, 25*(2), 149–152.

Lancioni, G. E., Connix, F., Manders, N., & Driessen, M. (1989). Use of automatic cueing to reduce drooling in two multihandicapped students. *Journal of the Multihandicapped Person, 2*(3), 201–210.

Rapp, D. (1980). Drool control: Long-term follow-up. *Developmental Medicine and Child Neurology, 22*(4), 448–453.

Thomas-Stonell, N., & Greenberg, J. (1988). Three treatment approaches and clinical factors in the reduction of drooling. *Dysphagia, 3*(2), 73–78.

Thorbecke, P. J., & Jackson, H. J. (1982). Reducing chronic drooling in a retarded female using a multi-treatment package. *Journal of Behavior Therapy and Experimental Psychiatry, 13*(1), 89–93.

CHAPTER

Technology and Saliva Overflow

Learning Outcomes

- *Increase your awareness of current technological approaches to saliva overflow*

- *Become familiar with technology assessment tools: the Saliva Assessment Instrument, the Chin Dry System, and the Swallow Frequency Device*

- *Understand the research approaches to designing and applying technology to saliva overflow*

Assistive technology refers to the mechanical aids used to enhance the physical functions of a person's body. Assistive technology has existed in various forms for years, and current advances in technology have enabled researchers to develop new devices that improve the lives of the most physically disabled persons (Gray, Quatrano, & Lieberman, 1998). The term *assistive technology* should be defined in two parts to be understood properly. *Assistive* means helping, supporting, and aiding in accomplishing practical functions, tasks, or purposes for persons of all ages. *Technology* means reliance on simple as well as potentially highly complex tools, devices, and equipment (King, 1999).

People with disabilities have abilities as well as disabilities. People with disabilities might choose to use assistive technology in an effort to compensate for their limitations. Assistive technology provides them the opportunity to focus on participating fully in school, the workplace, or the community.

In the past decade, various technologies and assessment instruments have been developed to assist in managing saliva overflow for children with disabilities. In an effort to make more precise decisions about treatments and interventions, and to objectively quantify saliva production, several researchers have attempted to measure salivary output and overflow. This research has resulted in the development of internal and external saliva collection devices used to quantify saliva.

The frequency at which one swallows significantly affects the condition of saliva overflow, and swallow frequency varies from person to person and activity to activity. The frequency of a swallow is critical information to know about a person who drools, because there is a direct correlation between nonswallowing and the condition of saliva overflow. Different activities such as talking, reading, sleeping, and eating alter the number of times a person swallows per hour. For example, the number of times that a person swallows while eating is substantially higher than the number of times a person swallows while sleeping.

Various ways of quantifying the frequency of swallowing have been proposed. Researchers have discovered that the swallowing sound could be differentiated from other sounds such as talking and coughing and thus the swallow sound could be counted (see Table 7.1). Lear, Flanagan, and Moorrees (1965, pp. 86–87) discovered that "when swallowing, a short sharp noise was invariably detectable with a stethoscope on the skin lateral to the laryngeal prominence." Lear et al. used simple equipment that was able to collect the sound of a swallow of the research participants for long periods of time. A small hearing aid microphone was attached to a participant's neck and then connected to the recorder microphone with tapes that recorded sounds for 8½ hours.

SALIVA COLLECTION TOOLS

Saliva Collection Inside the Mouth

Over the years, saliva has been collected for research purposes, so scientists developed various saliva collection appliances that are placed inside the mouth. Typical saliva collection systems consist of an apparatus to collect the saliva, a suction device, and a saliva storage chamber. Most saliva collection devices have concentrated on collecting submandibular, sublingual, or parotid saliva in which one type of saliva is segregated from the other. It has not been the intent of past researchers to collect the saliva to free the person of unwanted saliva.

Wolff, Begleiter, and Moskona (1997) developed a saliva collection system in which submandibular/sublingual (sm/sl) saliva samples were collected directly into a storage tube for study and testing. This saliva collection device collected saliva accurately with respect to saliva collection values reported by developers of similar devices. Cannulation (inserting a small tube into the gland) of the submandibular and sublingual glands, which is more invasive than simply collecting the saliva, is an alternative method to collect sm/sl saliva.

Saliva Collection Outside the Mouth

Although no longer in use, the Chin Cup, developed by Sochaniwskyj (1982), collected and quantified saliva from a saliva overflow spill. The Chin Cup, which was custom fit to the user's chin, was handmade from San-Splint (a pliable type of plasterlike material). A

TABLE 7.1
Activities and Swallowing Frequency

Sleeping	7.5 swallows/hour
Eating	296 swallows/hour
Supine	31.4 swallows/hour
Reading	36.5 swallows/hour

Note. From "The Frequency of Deglutition in Man," by C. S. C. Lear, J. B. Flanagan, and C. F. A. Moorrees, 1965, *Archives of Oral Biology, 10*, pp. 83–99. Copyright 1965 by Elsevier Science. Reprinted with permission.

tight-fitting lid was attached to the cup, and the cup was held firmly but comfortably against the chin of the user. Slender, flexible, narrow plastic evacuation tubing was attached to the base of the Chin Cup and to a vacuum generator pump that evacuated the saliva collected in the cup. The vacuumed saliva was stored in a collection chamber that housed test tubes that measured the volume of the saliva. The Chin Dry System also uses external saliva collectors as described in detail in the following section.

Intraoral Saliva Collection Appliances

Brown et al. (2001) are currently developing an intraoral dental appliance that removes saliva.[1] Using a customized dental impression, a dental appliance is custom fit for the person who drools.

The appliance has a stainless steel tube that exits the mouth and is attached to a thin flexible silicon tube that is attached to a vacuum pump and saliva storage container. The vacuum apparatus is a modified version of the Chin Dry System (see following section). Thus far, with 6 research participants, it appears that the intraoral vacuuming appliance holds great promise for keeping the user totally dry.

ASSESSMENT TOOLS

Recently developed saliva assessment tools include the Saliva Assessment Instrument, the Chin Dry System,[2] and the Swallow Frequency Device.

Saliva Assessment Instrument

The Saliva Assessment Instrument is a standardized, comprehensive, semiquantitative measurement and evaluation tool for assessing a client's saliva overflow condition (Allaire & Marshall, 2000; see saliva overflow Web site, http://ihs.airweb.net). The caregiver and the clinician see four schematic drawings of individuals with saliva control problems of increasing severity, progressing from mild to moderate to severe to profuse (see Figure 7.1). Each respondent marks the drawing that most resembles the client's drooling pattern. The client, the caregiver, and the clinician find this method to be more objective than making a judgment about the level of drooling severity.

The Saliva Assessment Instrument consists of six parts. Part I deals with demographics of the client and provides an interview format of the client and caregiver's perception of the drooling problem. Perceptions sometimes differ depending on the responder. Part II allows for identifying typical seating and positioning and provides correct positioning scenarios for the client. Part III is the semiquantitative schematic drawing of the four different drooling scenarios that were described earlier. The caregiver, and when appropriate, the client, and the clinician determine which scenario best fits the client. Again there might be a difference of opinion among the three. Part IV comprises a checklist for the oral structure and function of the client's mouth including mobility of the tongue and lips. Part V determines the client's problem-solving ability for clues on cognitive functioning. Part VI is a log for the caregiver to take home for a week to track and assess the severity of the drooling condition. In addition to the frequency of spills, whether the spill is mild, moderate, severe, or profuse also is recorded.

---

[1] Research in progress funded by the U.S. Department of Health and Human Services, National Institutes of Health, National Institute of Dental and Craniofacial Research, grant number 143DE13635-01A1. The views expressed in this chapter do not necessarily reflect the opinion of the National Institutes of Health.
[2] U.S. Patent No. 5,980,498, 11/99; No. 09/565,169, 5/00.

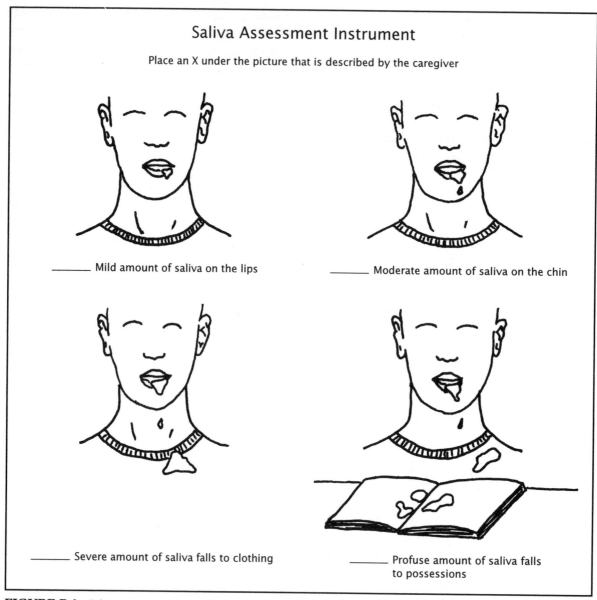

FIGURE 7.1. Saliva assessment instrument pictures.

Chin Dry System

Since 1996, researchers from Innovative Human Services, Inc., in collaboration with Allaire Development Company and Texas Scottish Rite Hospital for Children, of Dallas, Texas, have conducted research funded by the National Institutes of Health[3] titled *Technology for Swallowing Dysfunction and Sialorrhea: The Chin Dry System* (U.S. Department of Health and Human Services, 1996). The Chin Dry System technology helps people with saliva overflow to stay clean from unwanted saliva and its unpleasant side effects. The Chin Dry System is a functional hygienic device also designed for research and

---

[3] Authorization for this research is under grant number 5R44HD33300-03. The views expressed in this chapter do not necessarily reflect the opinion of the National Institutes of Health.

training. This device vacuums unwanted saliva and stores it for disposal (see Figures 7.2 and 7.3). By collecting the saliva, the user stays dry. The collected saliva also allows researchers to determine if attempted interventions result in less saliva being spilled. Saliva collection is done with noninvasive vacuum collectors that are worn on the shirt-front, are handheld, or are adhered to the chin (see Figure 7.4). The Chin Dry System monitors head tilt position while swallowing activity is monitored by the Swallow Frequency Device. The head tilt monitor and Swallow Frequency Device provide behavioral feedback to remind the user to hold their head up or to swallow. It also records and provides data to clinicians about these activities.

The Innovative Human Services, Inc., research team consulted with 29 consumer research participants and their caretakers about the design, function, benefits, and disadvantages of the Chin Dry System. The consumers used and manipulated the Chin Dry System saliva collectors while researchers noted what design changes were needed. Based on this intense feedback, the final Chin Dry System prototype was built and field-tested with 8 research participants (Brown & Allaire, 2000).

Field testing had two purposes. The first purpose was to determine if the Chin Dry System correctly detected the presence of a saliva spill and appropriately vacuumed and stored saliva for disposal. The second purpose was to determine if the research participants stayed drier when using the Chin Dry System than when not using it. The participants, all with cerebral palsy, were students in the Texas public schools. Four of the participants were male and 4 were female, ranging in age from 7 to 18 years. Seven of 8 participants were severe to profuse droolers, whereas the 8th participant was a moderate drooler. Participants were evaluated for severity of their saliva overflow problem and criteria were set for how wet or dry they were due to saliva overflow. Using single-subject

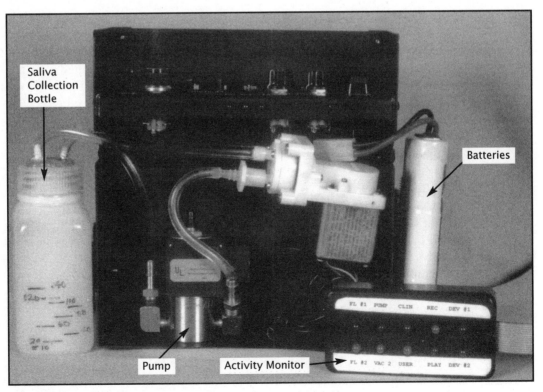

FIGURE 7.2. Chin Dry System.

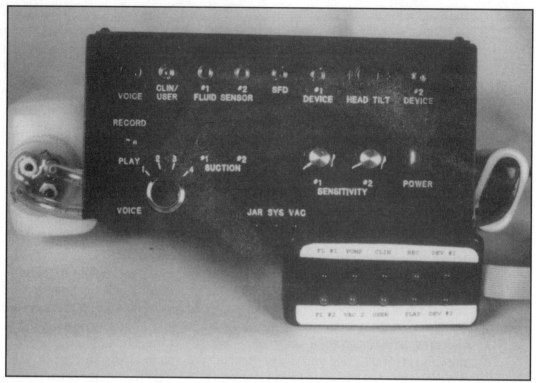

FIGURE 7.3. Top panel of the Chin Dry System.

ABAB designs, participants were evaluated for wetness or dryness while not using the Chin Dry System and then while using the Chin Dry System.

The Chin Dry System helped participants with saliva overflow to stay clean of unwanted saliva on the chin, shirtfront, and lap. It was determined that the Chin Dry System is effective and, in most cases, aesthetically acceptable. The shirtfront collector was effective, the easiest to use, and the most functional. The handheld collector was effective, but participants tired of having to pay attention and to consciously use the collector. The face collector was effective but least acceptable because it adhered to the chin and participants objected to being "messed with."

Swallow Frequency Device

Many sounds produced by the human pharynx and larynx are found to differ from one another by only 100 to 200 Hz. Previous researchers who have tried to isolate the swallow signal have used a frequency filter. But few devices are sensitive enough to distinguish between frequencies only 100 Hz apart. In response to this, Allaire Development Company in Charlottesville, Virginia, developed the Swallow Frequency Device, a noninvasive method for detecting swallowing behavior (Allaire, Allaire, & Baloh, 1999). The Swallow Frequency Device is an independent but also integrated component of the Chin Dry System. The Swallow Frequency Device is composed of a small stethophone that weighs less than a gram and a microprocessor that counts swallowing. The stethophone is fabricated from a stethoscope and a microphone in one unit (1.0 inch in diameter) that allows for optimum sound sensing. The stethophone is connected to a microprocessor and designed to record the sound pattern of a swallow.

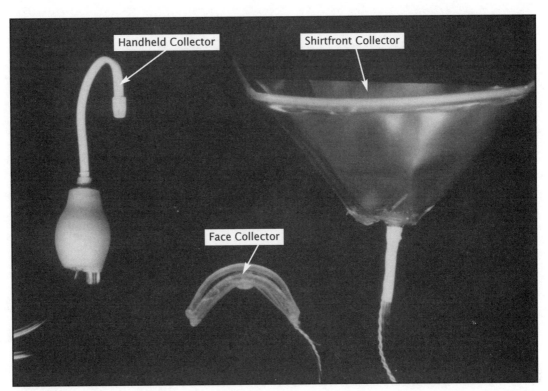

FIGURE 7.4. Saliva collectors.

Attachment of the stethophone to a reliable and valid position on the throat has been studied. Types of adhesives and methods of attachment have been tried with the optimum attachment protocol identified. Placement of the microphone on the throat has been investigated by using a gridlike frame on the throat (Takahashi, Groher, & Michi, 1994) and placing the stethophone to the right center of the cricoid-thyroid process. Using a type of sound-recognition software, an individual voluntarily swallows, coughs or speaks with the Swallow Frequency Device registering and disregarding these sounds. The Swallow Frequency Device recognizes the registered sounds, counts the number of swallows, and displays this count on the Swallow Frequency Device's digital screen. Currently in its fourth iteration (SFD4-OKI), the Swallow Frequency Device uses a microprocessor selected for its ability to learn and recognize sound patterns such as swallows, while rejecting other sounds such as speech.

The SFD4-OKI employs a digital time-domain electronic filter that is designed, because of the repeatability of swallow sounds made by individuals, to recognize the particular swallow frequency and amplitude and to reject all other foreign frequencies and amplitudes. The frequencies are coordinated over a time domain. Testing is ongoing for adaptability of the characteristics of the SFD4-OKI and its software.

Dedication to developing new technologies assists people with disabilities to overcome some of their limitations. In the field of sialorrhea research, a variety of technologies to control drooling have appeared within the past few decades, with some being more or less effective and invasive than others. The integration of technologies into studying solutions for people with saliva overflow difficulties has created a new field of interesting possibilities. So far there has been limited, but promising, success.

REFERENCES

Allaire, J. H., Allaire, P. E., & Baloh, M. (1999, June). *Swallow Frequency Device: A method of swallow detection.* Proceedings of the 20th Annual Conference of RESNA, Long Beach, CA.

Allaire, J. H., & Marshall, D. (2000, June). *The Saliva Assessment Instrument.* Proceedings of the 21st Annual Conference of RESNA, Orlando, FL.

Brown, C. C., & Allaire, J. (2000, March). *The Chin Dry System and the Swallow Frequency Device: A four-year research study of technologies for saliva overflow and swallowing problems.* Proceedings of the 15th Annual CSUN Conference, Los Angeles, CA.

Brown, C. J., Richardson, S., Inga, C., Allaire, J. A., Atkinson, J. A., & Trent, L. (2001). *An intraoral saliva-vacuuming appliance.* Unplublished report.

Gray, D. B., Quatrano, L. A., & Lieberman, M. L. (1998). *Designing and using assistive technology: The human perspective.* Baltimore: Brookes.

King, T. W. (1999). *Assistive technology: Essential human factors.* Boston: Allyn & Bacon.

Lear, C. S. C., Flanagan, J. B., & Moorrees, C. F. A. (1965). The frequency of deglutition in man. *Archives of Oral Biology, 10,* 83–99.

Sochaniwskyj, A. (1982). Drool quantification: Noninvasive technique. *Archives of Physical and Medical Rehabilitation, 63,* 605–607.

Takahashi, K., Groher, M. E., & Michi, K. (1994). Methodology for detecting swallowing sounds. *Dysphagia, 9,* 54–62.

U.S. Department of Health and Human Services, National Institutes of Health, National Institute of Child Health and Human Development, National Institute of Rehabilitation Research (1996).

Wolff, A., Begleiter, A., & Moskona, D. (1997). A novel system of human submandibular/sublingual saliva collection. *Journal of Dental Research, 76,* 1782–1786. *Technology for swallowing dysfunction and sialorrhea: The Chin Dry System.* Washington, DC: Author.

CHAPTER

Intraoral Appliances for Saliva Control

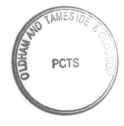

Learning Outcomes

■ *Name two different oral appliances*

■ *List the advantages and disadvantages of using an oral appliance*

■ *Explain why postural therapy is an integral part of appliance therapy*

■ *Understand the importance of the team approach*

Abnormal muscle tone and movement of the tongue, lips, and cheeks often results in changes to oral structures and consequent difficulty attaining functional oral movements, such as lip closure, voluntary tongue movement, chewing, and swallowing. Various intraoral appliances have been developed in an attempt to modify and improve oral–motor function. These appliances vary in the shape, the methods of attachment within the oral cavity, and the length of time they remain in the mouth. Appliances have been used with people with developmental as well as acquired disabilities (Asher & Winquist, 1994; Moulding & Koroluk, 1991). The use of oral appliances should be seen as part of a holistic approach that includes postural control of the whole body. Intraoral appliances are well accepted in Europe (Gisel, Schwartz, & Haberfellner, 1999a; Limbrock, Hoyer, & Scheying, 1990) as an integral part of oral–motor therapy. The most appropriate clinical population for these appliances are people with moderate impairments of the oral–motor system. The effects of therapy with these appliances are increased tongue mobility, improved resting posture of the tongue and lips, and improved sensation of the oral cavity. These changes result in improved oral transport followed by marked improvement in swallowing and decreased drooling.

These devices need a dentist or suitably qualified personnel to ensure the appliances fit correctly. Regular checks of the mouth and appliance also mean that the family, caregiver, and person using the appliance will need to visit the dentist regularly.

Saliva control has rarely been the primary aim of clinical trials of oral appliances in general and has been researched infrequently. For the appliances discussed in this chapter, however, a reduction in drooling has been reported in the literature.

When the use of an appliance for the purpose of saliva control is contemplated, the following considerations need to be addressed:

- the person's ability to retain the appliance securely, which may vary because of dentition, oral muscle tone, intraoral sensation, overall postural control, cooperation, and comfort;

- the person's motivation and ability to comply with the program;

- the availability of regular support and review by appropriate dental or orthodontic staff;

- the caregiver's willingness to support the therapy over a long period of time; and

- the person's physiological and behavioral ability to tolerate the appliance. (The person must be able to breathe easily through the nose while the appliance is in place.)

Some of the advantages and disadvantages of appliances for saliva control are presented in Table 8.1.

APPLIANCES AS PART OF A HOLISTIC APPROACH

The muscular connections of the bony structures of the head, neck, and shoulder girdle are often neglected with respect to the rest of the body, but there are multiple linkages throughout the body that can have positive and negative effects on facial and oral function. Economy is the major positive factor of this arrangement because a small number of structures can be used for many functions. Dysfunctions of the lips, tongue, palate, and pharynx are often seen as local problems. In fact these problems are frequently caused by postural inadequacy of the trunk, especially the neck and limbs. The complex structural and functional interrelations result in very different pathologic conditions that

TABLE 8.1
Advantages and Disadvantages of Using Oral Appliances for Saliva Control

Advantage	Disadvantage
Noninvasive (i.e., it does not involve drugs or anesthesia)	May be difficult to take a dental impression
The person has control over the wearing of the appliance	Needs regular visits to the dentist
Can result in long-term improvements	Can be expensive, because a number of visits to the dentist are needed
Usually temporary therapy	Cannot be worn if the person has nasal obstructions
Increases dental hygiene	Needs a skilled team experienced in this area
Involves a team approach	Needs careful evaluation
Can also improve eating and drinking skills	Appliance may break (usually happens outside the mouth) and need fixing

show striking similarities of facial and oral appearance. Although the relationship between oral dysfunction and postural impairment is readily observed in different forms of cerebral palsy, the same principle applies to other conditions. These conditions include simple developmental delay, enlarged adenoids, muscular or spinal diseases, Moebius syndrome, and pseudobulbar palsy.

Diverse conditions can be treated effectively if certain key issues are not ignored. These issues include maintaining the optimal posture of the whole body, down to the fingers and toes, and an awareness of the reciprocal (bidirectional) influences from the neck to the whole body, including the oral region (Crickmay, 1966; Finnie, 1974). For most people, the feeling of security and stability is a prerequisite to feeling comfortable. Open, clear, and unambiguous communication between the person and the therapist is extremely important.

THE TEAM AND THE ASSESSMENT OF THE PATIENT

Oral appliances are part of a combined therapeutic approach that involves all members of the team that is composed of rehabilitation physicians, speech–language pathologists, physical therapists, and dentists or orthodontists. It is important that postural control of the shoulder girdle, neck, and trunk are addressed as an integral background to therapy. Each member of the team has a specific role and needs an understanding of the roles and expertise of the other team members.

ASSESSMENT

The assessment should be done in a clinic designated for oral–motor disabilities by a team of pediatricians, developmental neurologists or rehabilitation doctors, orthodontists or dentists, and all therapists who work on oral problems (speech–language pathologists, occupational therapists, physical therapists). The child or adult and his or her family are also an integral part of the team.

The usual neurological examination rarely reveals the actual motor potential of the lips, cheeks, tongue, and velopharynx for oral transport. For the actual motor potential to be revealed, the techniques developed by oral therapists to assist the patient with postural control of all body parts need to be applied (Crickmay, 1966; Morris & Dunn-Klein, 2000; Mueller, 1974; Nelson, Meek, & Moore, 1994; Wolf & Glass, 1992). It is important that the team includes members experienced in the use of such assistive techniques.

An assessment of the individual's eating and drinking is important to display his or her full oral potential. Because eating and drinking are often seen as motivating and familiar activities, this assessment should not prove difficult. Food that might challenge the oral structures can assist in assessing a child's eating potential. Thus, solid bread including the crusts or slices of apple and (assisted) drinking from a cup will demonstrate the oral potential. Care must be taken to ensure that choking does not occur, and good postural handling techniques are necessary. Liquid and soft consistencies are not as helpful during the assessment process, because these will only produce midline movements (mostly of an oscillating character). The evaluation of eating and drinking, together with observations from the speech–language pathologist, guides the clinical indications for appliance therapy. This evaluation also will assist the construction of the device to best meet the needs of the individual.

Treatment goals concerning drooling, mouth closure, facial expression, eating and drinking, competence, and speech are discussed and decided on at the beginning of appliance therapy by the patient and caregiver. The team includes the patient and caregiver when deciding on the treatment goals. The idea is to stop therapy when goals are achieved.

Therapies, sports, and the correct use of equipment can improve oral functions because they all assist the patient with postural control of the body. Particularly useful therapeutic sports include swimming (Lambeck & Stanat, 2000) and riding on horseback. But note that even well-adapted seating or splints or body suits cannot be taken as ready solutions. They have to be reviewed regularly.

ORAL APPLIANCES

There have been a number of appliances developed over the years, including the palatal training appliance (PTA) and the vestibular screen, but the most commonly used appliances are the Castillo-Morales palatal plates and the Innsbruck Sensori Motor Activator and Regulator (ISMAR).

PTA

This appliance was first developed in England and was designed initially for people with hypernasal speech (Tudor & Selley, 1974; see Figure 8.1). It also was found to improve swallowing performance and to decrease drooling (Selley, 1977).

The device is made from a loop of stainless steel wire that is bent into a U shape and made to conform to the vault of the resting soft palate. It does not touch the soft palate but touches the mucous membrane near the base of the uvula. It is worn on an acrylic plate or fitted to a denture. The wire loop is adjustable and needs to be securely fitted to prevent it from being swallowed by clients who have reduced palatal sensitivity. The device is worn during the day but removed during sleep. An initial increase in salivation was reported. This increase was followed within a month by an increased rate of swallowing.

It has been suggested that the PTA works by increasing tactile awareness or by adding an extra stimulus to trigger involuntary swallowing (increasing the stimulus to the afferent side of the reflex arc to the swallowing center). The PTA also has been used to assist with swallowing in infants (Selley & Boxall, 1986). The loop in these cases was 0.7 mm, and a dental plate was made to fit the baby's upper jaw. It is to be worn all the time until swallowing improves.

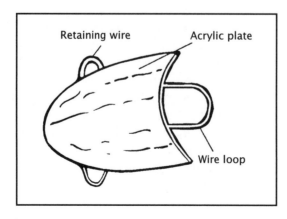

FIGURE 8.1. Palatal training appliance.

The Vestibular Screen

This is an acrylic device that sits between the lips and the teeth in the anterior vestibulum (see Figure 8.2). It is designed to encourage lip closure. Vestibular screens can be individually designed but also are commercially available. The therapy can be active or passive. If active therapy is used, the person sits with the vestibular screen in the buccal cavity with the lips purposively closed. The person should be instructed to hold on to the screen with his or her lips. Therapeutic exercises may assist the development of lip strength by the person's partner pulling on the vestibular shield's protruberance centrally and then laterally to encourage the orbicularis oris muscles to work. Passive use of the device can be achieved by wearing it at night when the person is asleep. Here the device assists with lip closure and an improved tongue position in a subconscious manner.

Castillo-Morales Appliances

The Castillo-Morales appliances were developed by using the principles of the Orofacial Regulation Therapy, which was designed in the 1970s for children with Down syndrome. Castillo-Morales, Limbrock, and others have modified the appliance to assist in the care of children with cerebral palsy to improve their oral–motor functions (Fischer-Brandies, Avalle, & Limbrock, 1987; Hohoff & Ehmer, 1999; Hoyer & Limbrock, 1990; Limbrock, Fischer-Brandies, & Avalle, 1991; Sjögreen, 2001; Wells, 2000). The fitting of stimulatory plates was undertaken concurrently with an exercise program based on physical therapy and speech–language therapy. The plate consists of a removable orthodontic plate with different stimulators placed to activate the required response. It is suggested that when there is a forward placement of the tongue, best results are achieved by a buttonlike stimulator at the dorsal edge of the plate, which must have a deep central hole to induce a sucking effect on the back of the tongue while pressed against the button. To correct an asymmetry of the tongue or a restricted lateral movement, the stimulator can be adjusted to the left or the right. To activate the upper lip movement, the plate has deeply grooved lip stimulators or mobile beads mounted on a vestibular wire similar to the ISMAR. Limbrock et al. (1990) consider that when the plate is worn for periods of an hour or half hour at a time through the day for 4 hours total, but not during sleep, there was an improvement of 72% in severe drooling. There have been no studies with randomized control groups, which could be considered a limitation of the evaluation of efficacy.

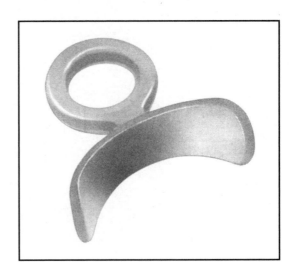

FIGURE 8.2. Vestibular screen. Copyright 2001 by Dr. F. G. Sand. Reprinted with permission.

CASE STUDY

James is a 5-year-old boy with a developmental disability. He presented with an open mouth posture, incompetent lip, severe drooling, and an inability to lateralize his tongue when eating.

After 3 months of neuromuscular facilitation and behavioral therapy, his drooling problem resolved, which also coincided with having decayed teeth removed. An oral appliance was used to encourage lip closure and lateral tongue movements. The appliance has a passive labial arch bar with stimulators to encourage lip closure. An active palatal lateral bar with moveable ring to stimulate lateral tongue movements also was added.

After 3 months of use 30 minutes twice daily, he could execute lateral tongue movements more frequently and with less difficulty, and he could attain lip closure with more ease. The appliance has been inserted, and the effect on lip posture is evident.

ISMAR

The ISMAR is an individually tailored combination of two classical orthodontic devices: the Andresen-Haeupl monobloc activator, itself a modification of P. Robin's monobloc, and the Fraenkel Regulator (see Figures 8.3 and 8.4). Despite the ISMAR's appearance, it is not an orthodontic device but aims at the sensorimotor improvement of facial, oral, and pharyngeal structures. An ISMAR is worn primarily to achieve jaw stabilization and, secondarily, to activate and mobilize the oral and pharyngeal structures.

ISMARs are considered to improve the oral posture and stimulate not only movements of lips, cheeks, and tongue but also the velopharynx indirectly. They are different from other oral devices in that they offer an opportunity for the individual to directly and actively stabilize the mandible and the hyoid bone, which in turn gives the necessary proximal stability to the tongue to allow voluntary movements of the tongue tip. This movement is comparable to the minimal amount of "mobile stability" of the neck, trunk, shoulder girdle, and arm that is needed to allow coordination of fine finger movements. If the person does not "grip" the ISMAR actively but leaves it loosely in the mouth, other important aspects of learning become possible. Voluntary or even involuntary

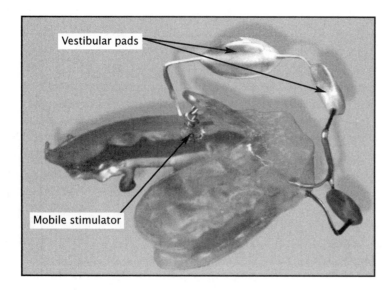

FIGURE 8.3. Innsbruck Sensori Motor Activator and Regulator. *Note.* Copyright 2000 by H. Haberfellner. Reprinted with permission.

FIGURE 8.4. Innsbruck Sensori Motor Activator and Regulator. *Note.* Copyright 2000 by H. Haberfellner. Reprinted with permission.

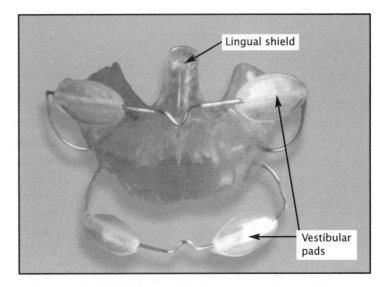

movements of the tongue will affect the monobloc component of the ISMAR, which will in turn move the vestibular pads. The person can then monitor involuntary tongue movements and the following lip movements and also the opposite sequence. It is possible to gradually learn to change these movements. Thus, the ISMAR must never be fixed in the mouth.

CASE STUDY

Matthias has an ataxia and a spastic diplegia. At 5 years of age, he commenced wearing a vestibular screen and at 6 years he changed to an ISMAR. He had habitually retracted lips, very restricted lip and tongue movements, drooling, and poor speech. By the time he was 7 years old, he was showing moderate improvements in lip position, tongue movements, chewing, and drooling. He also had stopped tooth grinding and coughing during meals. Over the next few years, his salivary control varied. Around puberty, his epileptic fits were especially hard to control. After 8 years of ISMAR use, all therapy goals had been achieved, and he no longer drooled. What also was impressive were the improvements in his facial expression and articulation. He has maintained these changes for the past 20 years.

Changing the engagement of the teeth and gums of the lower and upper jaws on the lateral occlusal shelves of the monobloc portion of the ISMAR can teach the person to grade mandibular stabilization (Gisel, Haberfellner, & Schwartz, 1999b, 2001; Haberfellner, 1992). Such stabilization of the tongue base alone without any further stimulation will allow some patients to move the tongue tip. These movements can be seen through the transparent anterior-medial tongue shield, which is the central and upwardly extended part of the monobloc portion. The tongue (lingual) shield is to prevent tongue thrust and further to alter lingual shape and position to ease swallowing.

During therapy, immobile and later mobile stimulators for lips or tongue and pharynx are introduced according to the patient's progress. All parts of the device, including the lingual as well as the vestibular stimulators, are large at the beginning of therapy.

This is irrespective of whether people are hypersensitive, hyposensitive, or have uncontrolled jaw movements.

 CASE STUDY

Alfred had athetosis resulting from an untreated severe neonatal hyperbilirubinaemia, but he had learned to walk. Until he was 7 years old, he underwent traditional neurodevelopment treatment. He commenced with the ISMAR at 8 years of age. At this time, he presented with an extremely protruding tongue (his parents had twice refused suggestions of a tongue-reduction operation) and profuse drooling. He could only bite and was unable to chew. He was retching at mealtimes, although he was hyposensitive inside his mouth. Four years later (at 12 years of age), he had no drooling and had a normal facial appearance. Eating and drinking were completely normal, as was his speech, whether face-to-face or on the telephone. Now at 35 years of age, he works as a hospital administrator with normal oral functions.

In the construction of the appliance, impressions are necessary for the production of the device. It is advisable to have the therapist or caregiver with the patient on the dental chair, especially if the patient is very young or has severe sensorimotor involvement (Gisel et al., 1999). It is important to prepare the child to cooperate in taking the impressions, because general anesthesia is not used.

The construction bite (registration of the jaws) is difficult to obtain intraorally in many cases. Consequently, the stone models are handheld and put into optimal intercuspidation. The mandible should be brought forward 1 to 2 mm and the bite opening should be 2 to 4 mm anteriorly and exceed the molar opening by 1 to 2 mm. Midline relations should be maintained. It is important not to cause significant displacement of the temporomandibular joint, and that the dentist or orthodontist assess and continually evaluate its status. It is also important that the appliance is constructed accurately, because adjustment before insertion can jeopardize success.

EVALUATION

There have been a number of studies that have assessed the value of intraoral appliances in different groups with different goals. Castillo-Morales, Grott, Avalle, and Limbrock (1982) investigated 59 Down syndrome patients by using their palatal plate, with the aims of increasing lip closure and reducing tongue protrusion. They found improvement in 49 patients. Similarly, Limbrock et al. (1990) studied 55 Down syndrome patients and found that 38 patients had decreased drooling.

Carlstedt, Dahllof, Nilsson, and Modeer (1996) studied the effect of palatal plate therapy on mouth closure in 14 children with Down syndrome compared with a control group of 15 children. The control group consisted of children with Down syndrome who received no treatment. There were statistically significant outcomes in closed mouth posture. This study was not measuring improvements in saliva control but noted "The parents in the treatment group reported improvements in eating and drinking habits and also less drooling" (p. 125).

In a pilot study, Haberfellner and Rossiwall (1977) found that 7 out of 9 patients showed marked or excellent improvement in normalizing oral sensitivity, lip seal, and saliva control using an ISMAR. Haberfellner (1981) attempted to circumvent the necessity of a control group by comparing improvements in oral dysfunction in a group of 20 children treated with a vestibular screen and 30 children treated with an ISMAR, while keeping all other therapeutic aspects identical. Three functions—oral sensitivity, lip mobility, and drooling—improved at about the same frequency but to a lesser degree than those in the ISMAR group. Gisel et al. (2001) used yet another approach with the functional assessment in 6-month time sequences and each person being her or his own control.

 ## CASE STUDY

Pauline is blind in her left eye and has very poor sight in her right eye, despite a series of operations beginning in the first weeks after birth. She has right-sided spastic hemiplegia. As a young person, she had difficulties eating and drinking. As her oral dysfunction became obvious, oral therapy was initiated, which included icing. Her drooling problem was not resolved. The use of a vestibular screen when she was around 10 years old did not help much either.

At the age of 19 years, she was about to leave her school and institution for the blind and partially sighted. Her voluntary lip and tongue movements were limited. She spoke slowly, hypernasally, and she could not pronounce some sounds such as L, R, S, and SH. She used computer facilities to scan in texts and convert them to Braille or make them audible by using speech synthetization that was available in 1987. Her trainers were reluctant to have her at the computer because she drooled (one to three times per hour, but it was more intensive when she was under stress, when she had a cold, and 2 premenstrual days), and they were concerned about her wetting the keyboard.

Further therapy was necessary, and in 3 weeks time she commenced wearing an ISMAR overnight. After 2 more months, her drooling was much improved. She could now wear the same sweater for 2 days, even in winter. For the first time, she also could be understood on the phone.

After 6 months, there was further improvement indicated by the first voluntary movements of her tongue to the side of her mouth. Twelve months later, she rarely retched when her tongue tip reached the lip border. Two years later, she was very confident in public, and although she spoke slowly her articulation was nearly perfect. She began to speak to unknown people on the phone. Her drooling ceased, and there were no longer any difficulties eating or drinking. She stopped using the ISMAR after 5 years at the age of 24 years. At the age of 30 years, there has been no deterioration in her oral skills. She works as an advertisement consultant and speaks slowly but with almost normal articulation.

REFERENCES

Asher, R. S., & Winquist, H. (1994). Appliance therapy for chronic drooling in a patient with mental retardation. *Special Care in Dentistry, 14*(1), 30–32.

Carlstedt, K., Dahllof, G., Nilsson, B., & Modeer, T. (1996). Effect of palatal plate therapy in children with Down syndrome. A 1-year study. *Acta Odontologica Scandinavica, 54*(2), 122–125.

Castillo-Morales, R., Grotti, E., Avalle, C., & Limbrock, G. (1982). Orofazial regulation beim Down-Syndrom durch Gaumenplatte. *Sozialpadiatrie, 4,* 10–17.

Crickmay, M. (1966). *Speech therapy and the Bobath approach to cerebral palsy.* Springfield, IL: Thomas.

Finnie, N. R. (1974). *Handling the young cerebral palsied child at home* (2nd ed.). London: Heinemann.

Fischer-Brandies, H., Avalle, C., & Limbrock, G. J. (1987). Therapy of orofacial dysfunctions in cerebral palsy according to Castillo-Morales: First results of a new treatment concept. *European Orthodontic Society, 9,* 139–143.

Gisel, E. G., Schwartz, S. T., & Haberfellner, H. (1999a). Impact of oral appliance (ISMAR) therapy: Are oral skills maintained 1 year after termination of therapy? [Scientific posters]. *Developmental Medicine and Child Neurology, 43.*

Gisel, E. G., Schwartz, S. T., & Haberfellner, H. (1999b, May/June). The Innsbruck Sensorimotor Activator and Regulator (ISMAR): Construction of an intraoral appliance to facilitate ingestive functions. *Journal of Dentistry for Children, 180–187.*

Gisel, E., Haberfellner, H., & Schwartz, S. (2001). Impact of oral appliance therapy: Are oral skills and growth maintained one year after termination of therapy? *Dysphagia, 16*(4), 296–307.

Haberfellner, H. (1981). Therapy of facio-oro-pharyngeal dysfunctions in cerebral palsied patients. *Neuropediatrics, 44,* 204–215.

Haberfellner, H. (1992, Spring). ISMAR: A rewarding co-operation of the dental profession with the rehabilitation teams for the treatment of disturbances of face, mouth and throat. *Interlink,* 4–6.

Haberfellner, H., & Rossiwall, B. (1977). Appliances for treatment of oral sensori–motor disorders. *American Journal of Physical Medicine, 56,* 5241–5248.

Hohoff, A., & Ehmer, U. (1999). Short-term and long-term results after early treatment with Castillo-Morales stimulating plate. *Journal of Orofacial Orthopedics Fortschritte der Kieferothopadie, 60,* 2–12.

Hoyer, H., & Limbrock, J. G. (1990). Orofacial regulation therapy in children with Down syndrome, using the methods and appliances of Castillo-Morales. *Journal of Dentistry for Children, 57,* 442–444.

Lambeck, J., & Stanat, F. (2000). The Halliwick concept. *Journal of Aquatic Physical Therapy, 8*(2), 6–11.

Limbrock, G. J., Fischer-Brandies, H., & Avalle, C. (1991). Castillo-Morales' orofacial therapy: Treatment of 67 children with Down syndrome. *Developmental Medicine and Child Neurology, 33*(4), 296–303.

Limbrock, G. J., Hoyer, H., & Scheying, H. (1990, November/December). Drooling, chewing and swallowing dysfunctions in children with cerebral palsy: Treatment according to Castillo-Morales. *Journal of Dentistry for Children,* 445–451.

Morris, S. E., & Dunn-Klein, M. (2000). Pre-feeding skills: A comprehensive resource for mealtime development (2nd ed.). San Antonio, TX: Psychological Corp.

Moulding, M. B., & Koroluk, L. D. (1991). An intraoral prosthesis to control drooling in a patient with amytrophic lateral sclerosis. *Special Care in Dentistry, 11*(5), 200–202.

Mueller, H. A. (1974). Feeding. In N. R. Finnie (Ed.), *Handling the young cerebral palsied child at home* (2nd ed., pp. 111–130). London: Heinemann.

Nelson, C. A., Meek, M. M., & Moore, J. C. (1994). *Head and neck treatment issues as a base for oral–motor function.* Albuquerque, NM: Clinician's View.

Selley, W. G. (1977). Dental help for stroke patients. *British Dental Journal, 143*(12), 409–412.

Selley, W. G., & Boxall, J. (1986). A new way to treat sucking and swallowing difficulties in babies. *The Lancet, I,* 1182–1184.

Sjögreen, L. (2001). Speech therapist in the orofacial treatment team. In M. Sillanpä (Ed.), *Practices on orofacial therapy* (pp. 11–15). Helsinki: Finnish Association of Orofacial Therapy.

Tudor, C., & Selley, W. G. (1974). A palatal training appliance and a visual aid for use in the treatment of hypernasal speech. A preliminary report. *British Journal of Disorders of Communication, 9,* 117–122.

Wells, R. (2000, August). Bonfire of love. *Exceptional Parent,* 40–44.

Wolf, L., & Glass, R. (1992). *Feeding and Swallowing disorders in infancy. Assessment and management.* San Antonio, TX: Psychological Corp.

Medical Management of Saliva

Learning Outcomes

- *List the principle types of drugs used in the management of secretions*

- *Outline the actions of these drugs*

- *Describe the factors that need to be taken into consideration when using these drugs*

- *Understand the role of botulinum and radiotherapy in the management of secretions*

A variety of medical interventions have been used in the medical management of salivary problems. Although all these methods have been found to be useful in some cases, all interventions have some drawbacks. There is a need for controlled clinical trials to examine issues concerning the suitability of particular patient groups and the appropriate dose and timing of individual types of intervention.

Individuals respond to salivary problems in different ways. For some people, a small amount of drooling is devastating, whereas others appear not to notice a severe drooling problem. The clinician must begin establishing the reactions and attitudes of the individual and all people involved in his or her care. For some individuals, the problem of drooling is socially distressing and can lead to self-imposed isolation. Other individuals, usually those with cognitive deficits, pay little attention to their drooling and the person's family or caregivers express concern about the problem. Problems associated with xerostomia also cause concern; however, because xerostomia is not visually obvious, there may be a tendency for caregivers and clinicians to be less aware of this problem, especially if the individual is unable to communicate easily (Smallwood, 1999).

EXCESS SECRETIONS AND DROOLING

Impaired spontaneous swallowing of saliva, poor lip control, or jaw muscle weakness can all result in the pooling of oral secretions and potential drooling, especially at mealtimes.

A range of drug treatments are used with the aim of reducing the flow of saliva by blocking the nerves stimulated by the autonomic nervous system by mechanical, sensory, or emotional stimuli (see Figure 9.1).

DRUGS THAT REDUCE SALIVA PRODUCTION

Anticholinergic Agents

propantheline bromide

hyoscine (scopolamine)

glycopyrrolate (Rubinol; Mier et al., 2000)

atropine sulphate

benzhexol (Artane; Reddihough, Johnson, Staples, Hudson, & Exarchos, 1990)

benztropine mesylate (Cogentin; Camp-Bruno, Winsberg, Green-Parsons, & Abrams, 1989)

tricyclic antidepressants, imipramine (Tofranil), amitriptyline (Tryptanol)

The most commonly used medications have anticholinergic properties that block the parasympathetic innervation of the salivary glands. The parasympathetic nerves regulate the secretion of the fluid component of saliva, therefore anticholinergic drugs primarily reduce the volume of saliva produced and have a lesser effect on the secretion of salivary proteins, the mucoid component.

These medications are usually given orally but scopolamine can be administered by using a transdermal patch (although there is difficulty obtaining these patches in some parts of the world). Other drugs (e.g., hyoscine, glycopyrrolate, atropine) can be given subcutaneously, which can be particularly useful in a palliative care setting.

Side Effects

Side effects of anticholinergic agents can include blurred vision, glaucoma, delayed gastric emptying, flushing, dry skin, tachycardia (palpitations), and confusion. Constipation

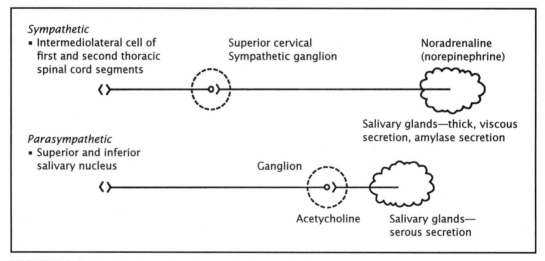

FIGURE 9.1. Model of neural mediation of saliva production.

and urinary retention are troublesome peripheral side effects of anticholinergic medication on the autonomic nervous system. Because of these side effects, doses for the elderly or patients with neurological disease that predisposes them to sphincter disturbance, such as multiple sclerosis or Parkinson's disease, should be closely monitored.

Some patients find the mouth-drying effect of anticholinergic agents uncomfortable. A reduction in salivary flow rates can result in thicker, more tenacious oral–pharyngeal secretions, which are difficult for patients with oral–pharyngeal weakness to spit out or swallow. The elderly, patients with dementia or other forms of cortical brain damage, and young children may poorly tolerate this type of medication and show with increased irritability and confusion. Patients with glaucoma should not be given anticholinergic medication unless under the supervision of an ophthalmologist.

Sympathomimetic Drugs and Antihistamines

pseudoephredrine
antihistamines

These drugs are usually found in combination in proprietary decongestant medications for colds and hay fever. In addition to blocking immune-mediated secretion from mucous membranes, antihistamines also produce mucosal drying through anticholinergic effects. Sympathomimetic agents reduce secretions by causing vasoconstriction within the mucous membranes.

Side Effects

Side effects of antihistamines include drowsiness and the anticholinergic side effects previously described. Sympathomimetic drugs should be avoided in patients with hypertension or hyperthyroidism, and they are contraindicated in patients taking monoamine oxidase inhibitor drugs for depression.

Adaption and Rebound

A problem that initially was well controlled with medication may return after a period of continuous medication. This problem of tachyphylaxis results from prolonged drug exposure (Korol, Sletten, & Brown, 1966). A related problem can occur if medication is suddenly stopped. The level of saliva output will have stabilized on the medication; cessation of the medication will lead to a marked increase in output because of induced hypersensitivity of the receptors in the salivary glands (Westlind-Danielsson, Muller, & Bartfai, 1990), which is known as "the rebound effect." For this reason, medication should be tapered off gradually when it is to be stopped.

MEDICATIONS THAT ALTER THE CONSISTENCY OF ORAL SECRETIONS

Sympathetic Nervous System Blocking Drugs

Parasympathetic nerve stimulation results in increased saliva flow with little salivary protein secretion, but animal studies indicate the opposite is achieved with stimulation of the sympathetic innervation of the salivary glands. Sympathetic adrenergic blocking agents, therefore, would not be expected to influence the amount of saliva formed but may affect its consistency.

It is not clearly understood how cholinergic, adrenergic, and peptidergic neurotransmitters are functionally integrated to modulate saliva production in response to various stimuli. The use of sympathetic receptor blocking agents is unproven in the treatment of saliva control problems.

Mucolytic Agents

citric acid

papaya extract

acetylcysteine

bromhexine

Thick, ropy secretions are difficult to spit out and may obstruct swallowing. Patients with this problem may already have a dry feeling in the mouth, and their symptoms are often made worse by the "drying" agents described previously. Mucolytic agents are aimed at breaking down the protein content of mucoid secretions. Citric acid in fruit juices and proteolytic enzymes such as papaya are good first-line therapy. Mucolytic drugs can be administered by inhalation (acetylcysteine) or orally (bromhexine). However, they can cause gastric irritation.

CHOICE OF DRUG AND INITIATION OF TREATMENT

The choice of medication will be guided by the clinical assessment of the individual patient, taking into consideration any contraindications to specific drugs as previously outlined. The assessment can be made more objective by observing the patient at various times of day. Diurnal variation in saliva control problems also can be reported subjectively by the patient using simple charts (see Assessment of Secretions, Chapter 3). Medication is not always effective in reducing saliva-related problems, and the dosage required for any individual is quite variable. This must be explained at the commencement of treatment. Side effects should be discussed carefully with individuals and their families.

All drugs should be commenced at the lowest dose, given once or twice daily, and increased gradually until optimum effectiveness or limited side effects occur. Intelligent timing of doses, along with knowledge of the half-life of the various drugs, will allow maximum benefit at problem times (e.g., meals, social occasions, bedtime). Unless side effects occur, each drug should be given an adequate trial at what is considered by the prescribing clinician to be a full therapeutic dose before being considered ineffective. The dose schedule attained and reasons for withdrawal of the drug should be well documented in the patient's records to guide future management.

Medication is not usually considered a long-term treatment option in the management of drooling in children. However, it is quite useful in a number of situations.

1. It can be used for short periods as an adjunct to behavioral methods, which may be easier to implement with a drier mouth.

2. Drooling may improve spontaneously in children up to the age of 6 to 7 years. Medication can be valuable in younger children when drooling causes major difficulty, allowing decisions about surgery to be deferred until later.

3. It can be used to assess the advantages of freedom from drooling before surgery is undertaken.

4. It has a role when drooling is a relatively minor problem. Individuals may use medication intermittently in situations in which drooling will pose a difficulty for them (e.g., social situations). One drug that may be used in this way is benzhexol hydrochloride. It begins to act within 1 hour, the peak effects last 2 to 3 hours, and the duration of action is 6 to 12 hours.

5. Medication may be used for severe drooling over an extended period in which (a) there has been a reluctance to undergo surgery, or (b) surgery is contraindicated (e.g., in older clients) or with individuals who have terminal conditions.

SUGGESTED PROTOCOLS FOR IMPLEMENTATION OF MEDICATION

Given clinicians' poor understanding of the complexity of the neural, humoral, and behavioral effects of saliva production and management, it is not surprising that available pharmacological agents can only imperfectly redress the imbalances that lead to saliva control problems. Accurate assessment and evaluation of response to treatment, therefore, help ensure the most appropriate application of limited therapeutic options.

Protocol 1. A protocol has been adopted for the use of benzhexol hydrochloride (Artane) in children older than the age of 3 years. The dosage is increased over a 6-week period. Drooling measurements are taken before medication and once the maximum dose has been reached.

1. The starting dose of benzhexol hydrochloride is 1 mg twice daily for 2 weeks.

2. If there is no improvement, the dose is increased to 2 mg twice daily for a further 2 weeks.

3. The dose may be further increased to a maximum dose of 2 mg three times daily.

Protocol 2. A protocol developed to assess the efficacy of medication prescribed to control oral secretions in adults uses an assessment form (refer to the Oral Secretion Assessment form in Appendix A). As well as documenting the presence of excessive amounts of saliva, this approach also addresses the consistency of the saliva and the daily pattern of the problem. This information helps guide the selection of medication and the timing of doses.

The individual's perception of the problem is discussed. The team members are taught how to use the form. Agreement is reached on how to interpret and quantify the various guidelines to be assessed. Follow-up assessments, using the same form, allow the person's response to dose increments to be monitored.

RADIATION

Xerostomia is a well recognized but unwanted side effect of radiation therapy to the head and neck, with the degree of xerostomia being related to the radiation dose. The use of radiation therapy in the management of drooling has received occasional attention in literature (Borg & Hirst, 1998). Improvements in the ability to control the dose and focus of X rays have rekindled interest in the use of radiotherapy to manage the problem of drooling. People with progressive diseases such as amyotrophic lateral sclerosis and Parkinson's disease have been considered appropriate for this method of management because it is relatively noninvasive, does not require an anesthetic, produces no surgical wound, and is quick and painless. Its use has the potential to reduce problems associated with medication and surgery. Considerations of possible radiotherapy-induced malignancies are less important because of the poor prognosis of people with these conditions.

The protocol outlined by Harriman et al. (2001) recommends a small single dose of radiation (8 Gy) be directed to the submandibular glands and the tail of the parotid. The submandibular gland is chosen as a main target of the treatment, rather than the parotid gland, because it produces most of the resting saliva. Resting saliva is considered to contribute more to the problem of drooling than saliva from the parotid glands. This is because saliva from the submandibular glands is produced throughout the day, and because it is not related to eating, the saliva is less likely to be swallowed and more likely to pool under the tongue and be drooled. Because in this protocol the parotid gland and minor salivary glands are relatively spared, the problems of dysphagia and poor oral health, secondary to xerostomia, are theoretically lessened.

Although radiotherapy appears to have the potential to be a valuable tool in the management of drooling, large multicenter evaluations of this technique are needed. Problems associated with xerostomia, poor oral health, and the return of salivary function have been noted, and these aspects need to be better documented.

BOTULINUM TOXIN

Another more recent addition to the range of treatments for drooling is the neurotoxin, botulinum, which has a record of effectiveness in autonomic disorders. Botulinum blocks the release of acetylcholine in the nerve terminals, at the neuromuscular junction, and also in the sympathetic and parasympathetic ganglion cells and in postganglionic parasympathetic nerves. Using a variety of assessment techniques, such as bib weighing, scintigraphy, and patient self-reporting, several researchers have found it to be effective in reducing the amount of saliva produced in the majority of patients (Bhatia, Munchau, & Brown, 1999; Giess et al., 2000; Jost, 1999; Pal, Calne, Calne, & Tsui, 2000; Porta, Gamba, Bertacchi, & Vaj, 2001; Winterholler, Erbguth, & Kat, 2001). However, at present, the use of botulinum for the reduction of salivary output is in a developmental phase, and several issues have been raised concerning its use.

The period of effectiveness has been found to vary between studies. Bhatia et al. (1999) reported that the response was maintained for 6 weeks to 4 months. Porta et al. (2001) reported that patients experienced a reduction in the saliva flow within 3 to 8 days after the injection and the response was maintained for 4 to 7 months.

It is still unclear which gland is the most appropriate for toxin injection, the most frequent choice being the parotid gland. This may be because the parotid gland is the easiest of the major salivary glands to access. Jost (1999) suggested that the parotid glands be injected first and then, if appropriate, the remaining major salivary glands should be injected. He considered this approach less risky because the parotid glands are anatomically further away from the pharyngeal musculature, which is responsible for airway protection during swallowing. The question remains as to whether the submandibular glands should be targeted first because they produce the majority of resting saliva, which is considered to be the source of most drooling. The actual placement of the botulinum injection is an important issue when considering the efficacy of this intervention. Bhatia et al.

(1999) reported weakness of the muscles of mastication following the injection of botulinum into the parotid glands. It was thought that this weakness might have been caused by the injection of botulinum into the surrounding tissue. Mezaki, Kaji, and Kohara (1996) raised the possibility of systemic absorption and distribution. They reported a case of generalized weakness in a woman with amyotrophic lateral sclerosis after a focal injection of botulinum.

In an attempt to restrict the botulinum to the salivary glands, Winterholler et al. (2001) adopted a transductal approach. This approach entailed injecting the botulinum directly into the gland via the salivary duct. However, they abandonded this technique because of the unwanted side effects of pain and inflamation of the treated glands.

Porta et al. (2001) addressed the issue of accurate placement of the injection by ultrasound to guide needle placement and reported an improvement in response, with all but one of the participants obtaining effective saliva reduction and only one case experiencing an unwanted outcome, marked xerostomia. This technique appears to offer a less invasive but temporary alternative approach to the reduction of saliva in people with drooling problems; however, further investigation is needed to refine the procedure.

REFERENCES

Bhatia, K. P., Munchau, A., & Brown, P. (1999). Botulinum toxin is a useful treatment in excessive drooling in saliva. *Journal of Neurology, Neurosurgery and Psychiatry, 67*(5), 697.

Borg, M., & Hirst, F. (1998). The role of radiation therapy in the management of sialorrhea. *International Journal of Radiation Oncology, Biology, Physics, 41*(5), 1113–1119.

Camp-Bruno, J. A., Winsberg, B. G., Green-Parsons, A. R., & Abrams, J. P. (1989). Efficacy of benztropine therapy for drooling. *Developmental Medicine and Child Neurology, 31*(3), 309–319.

Giess, R., Naumann, M., Werner, E., Riemann, R., Beck, M., Puls, I., Reiners, C., & Toyka, K. V. (2000). Injections of botulinum toxin A into the salivary glands improve sialorrhea in amyotrophic lateral sclerosis. *Journal of Neurology, Neurosurgery and Psychiatry, 69*(1), 121–123.

Harriman, M., Morrison, M., Hay, J., Ravonta, M., Eisen, A., & Lentle, B. (2001). Use of radiotherapy for control of sialorrhea in patients with amyotrophic lateral sclerosis. *Journal of Otolaryngology, 30,* 242–244.

Jost, W. G. (1999). Treatment of drooling in Parkinson's disease with botulinum toxin. *Movement Disorders, 14,* 1057.

Korol, B., Sletten, I. W., & Brown, M. L. (1966). Conditioned physiological adaptation to anticholinergic drugs. *American Journal of Physiology, 211*(4), 911–914.

Mezaki, T., Kaji, R., & Kohara, N. (1996). Development of generalized weakness in a patient with amyotrophic lateral sclerosis after focal botulinum toxin. *Neurology, 46*(3), 845–846.

Mier, R. J., Bachrach, S. J., Lakin, R. C., Barker, T., Childs, J., & Moran, M. (2000). Treatment of sialorrhea with glycopyrrolate. *Archives of Pediatrics and Adolescent Medicine, 154,* 1214–1218.

Pal, P. K., Calne, D. B., Calne, S., & Tsui, J. K. C. (2000). Botulinum toxin A as treatment for drooling saliva in PD. *Neurology, 54*(1), 244–247.

Porta, M., Gamba, M., Bertacchi, G., & Vaj, P. (2001). Treatment of sialorrhea with ultrasound guided botulinum toxin A injection in patients with neurological disorders. *Journal of Neurology, Neurosurgery and Psychiatry, 70*(4), 538–540.

Reddihough, D., Johnson, H., Staples, M., Hudson, I., & Exarchos, H. (1990). Use of benzhexol hydrochloride to control drooling of children with cerebral palsy. *Developmental Medicine and Child Neurology, 32*(11), 985–989.

Smallwood, S. (1999). *Problems with oropharyngeal secretions in Parkinson's disease.* Unpublished honor's thesis, Melbourne, Australia: La Trobe University.

Westlind-Danielsson, A., Muller, R. M., & Bartfai, T. (1990). Atropine treatment induced cholinergic supersensitivity at receptor and second messenger levels in the rat salivary gland. *Acta Physiologica Scandinavica, 138*(4), 431–441.

Winterholler, M. G. M., Erbguth, F. J., & Kat, S. (2001). Botulinum toxin for the treatment of siaalorrhea in ALS: Serious side effect of a transductal approach. *Journal of Neurology, Neurosurgery and Psychiatry, 70*(3), 417.

Surgical Management for Saliva Control

Learning Outcomes

■ *Recognize indications for surgical treatment of drooling*

■ *Outline the anatomical and physiological rationale for surgery*

■ *List the surgical procedures and various combinations of these procedures*

■ *Describe the results, complications, and pros and cons of different surgery approaches*

■ *Report on the approach used in Melbourne*

PRINCIPLES OF SURGERY FOR SIALORRHEA

The surgical management of drooling has been evolving for more than 30 years. The principles of surgery include planning a physiologically sound procedure with minimal changes to the environment of the mouth, minimal scarring and damage to the surrounding structures, and minimal risk of creating immediate, short-term, and long-term complications.

Indications for Surgical Treatment

There are several indicators that lead to the suggestion of a surgical approach. Usually there is a combination of factors and less invasive procedures are used initially. The indicators are as follows:

- Consider if the drooling is profuse and multiple changes of clothes or bibs during the day are needed. Conservative measures are unlikely to achieve a satisfactory outcome.

- Consider if the person has a severe physical or intellectual disability that affects his or her ability to follow instructions. Ethical issues need to be considered when the person with the disability is unable to provide informed consent.

- Consider if previous treatment, such as correction of situational factors (e.g., posture, nasopharyngeal obstruction, malocclusion), behavior modification, orofacial facilitation, appliances, and medication, has been unsuccessful. Even if these measures are unsatisfactory alone, they can assist with achieving a better surgical result in some cases.

- Consider if a child is older than 6 years of age. Maturation of orofacial function can continue at least up until the age of 6 years in developmentally delayed children.

Approximately one half of all patients presenting for salivary control management undergo surgery (Crysdale, Raveh, McCann, Roskee, & Aiona, 2001). In Melbourne, Australia, 96 of the 323 children who attended saliva clinics between 1986 and 2000 have had sialorrhea surgery.

SURGICAL OPTIONS

Potential surgical modalities include denervation of the salivary glands, excision of the salivary glands, ligation of salivary ducts, and relocation of ducts. The benefits of denervation are lost within a year, possibly as a result of reinnervation. Isolated salivary gland ablation, either by excision or duct ligation, may result in at least partial compensatory hypersecretion by residual salivary tissue. This partial compensatory hypersecretion has been demonstrated in the submandibular and parotid glands of rodents. Patients undergoing parotidectomy recently have been shown that their contralateral gland secretion increases by 30% under controlled conditions (Chaushu et al., 2001). This increase occurred in 10 of 17 patients. The increase was established within 3 weeks of surgery in those 6 patients with normal preoperative output. Four patients had compensated preoperatively because the disease process had already partially ablated parotid function. Seven of the 17 who were older and who had more advanced disease failed to compensate either pre- or postoperatively. Salivary amylase and electrolyte levels were unchanged in both glands. Alternative forms of treatment include temporary chemodenervation by intraglandular injections of botulinum toxin, radiotherapeutic ablation of salivary tissue function, and laser ablation of the parotid ducts, some of which have serious drawbacks.

The following paragraphs are brief descriptions of potential surgical modalities. A detailed description of the procedures and results follow.

1. *Parasympathectomy.* A transtympanic neurectomy can be used to interrupt the nerve supply to the parotid gland (tympanic plexus), as well as to the submandibular and sublingual glands (chorda tympani).

2. *Salivary gland excision.* The sublingual gland can be excised through an incision in the anterior aspect of the floor of the mouth, behind the teeth. The submandibular glands are excised through an external incision below the jaw. Parotid gland excision is carried out through an incision in front of and below the ear and involves dissection of the facial nerve, which is a major operation.

3. *Duct ligation.* The parotid duct can be ligated through a small incision on the inside of the cheek. This simple procedure, which can be carried out in about 5 minutes, results in an accumulation of saliva within the duct system, which results in some swelling within the firm parotid fascia. Back pressure causes secretion to cease and ultimately the gland becomes nonfunctional. Ligation of the submandibular duct has generally not been carried out because of the fear that the gland and floor of the mouth would swell, because this gland is not contained in a firm fibrous capsule as is the parotid gland. A recent small series of submandibular duct ligations sug-

gests that this can be a simple and efficacious way to ablate submandibular gland function (Klem & Mair, 1999), which has been confirmed in one case by the author of this chapter.

4. *Duct relocation*. The submandibular duct (Wharton's duct) can be transposed from its termination at the front of the tongue, behind the lower central incisors to the posterior part of the oral cavity, either in the tonsillar fossa or at the base of the tongue. This effective procedure in which an incision is made in the anterior floor of the mouth takes approximately 1 hour to perform. The parotid duct (Stenson's duct) can be elongated and transposed posteriorly (Wilkie, 1967). This surgery is no longer performed because of unacceptable morbidity.

Parasympathectomy (Transtympanic Neurectomy)

This surgery involves bilateral excision of the tympanic plexus and chorda tympani in the middle ear.

The parasympathetic fibers for the parotid originate in the inferior salivary nucleus of the brainstem and travel in the glossopharyngeal nerve (ninth) and then pass through the tympanic (Jacobson's) branch to the tympanic plexus. They then pass to the lesser superficial petrosal nerve to the otic ganglion just below the foramen ovale, where they then pass through the auriculotemporal branch of the trigeminal nerve (fifth) to the parotid gland. The submandibular and sublingual glands derive their parasympathetic fibers from the superior salivary nucleus. These fibers pass from the brain stem through the nervus intermedius of the facial nerve (seventh) through the chorda tympani to the lingual nerve branch of the trigeminal nerve (fifth). This nerve supplies the submandibular and sublingual glands through the submandibular ganglion. Nerve fibers supplying taste to the anterior two thirds of the tongue also pass through the nervus intermedius, chorda tympani, and lingual nerve.

Transtympanic neurectomy is performed bilaterally by reflecting the ear drum. The promontory should be drilled out to divide the hypotympanic branch of plexus. The chorda tympani is divided. Apart from loss of taste to the anterior two thirds of the tongue, there is little morbidity from this relatively simple otological procedure. It has been suggested that some children's diets "improved" in that they started to eat previously rejected foods such as cabbage. However, in general, patients do not become less interested in food nor is there any weight loss.

Crysdale (1980) reported that 20 of 33 patients improved after transtympanic neurectomy. Of the 13 cases that were not improved, some of these had unilateral procedures. Fourteen of 20 patients improved when complete neurectomy was performed bilaterally. There was a tendency for recurrence of drooling after 12 months, possibly due to reinnervation. This procedure was abandoned by Crysdale in favor of submandibular duct transpositions.

Parotid Duct Rerouting

Wilkie (1967) buried a tube of mucosa from parotid ducts into the tonsilla fossa with preliminary tonsillectomy. At a second operation, patients required submandibular gland excision. Wilkie and Brody (1977) reported good control in 90% of the patients, but 43 of 123 patients had complications, including wound breakdown, parotid duct stenosis, difficult oral hygiene, increased dental and gingival infections, and septic parotiditis.

Parotid Duct Ligation

Dundas and Peterson (1979) reported bilateral duct ligation with submandibular gland excision. Nine of 14 patients had good control and 2 had xerostomia. Crysdale had performed ligation in only 7 patients up until 1992. Varma, Henderson, and Cotton (1991) reported 14 cases of bilateral submandibular duct.

Submandibular Gland Excision

External neck incisions are required, which may result in unsightly scarring. This type of incision risks damage to the mandibular branch of the facial nerve, hypoglossal nerve, and lingual nerve.

Submandibular Duct Rerouting

This type of sugery was first reported by Ekedahl in 1974. In his 1980 paper, Crysdale, an ear, nose, and throat surgeon, suggested that these patients would often need a preliminary tonsillectomy and adenoidectomy. They required 1 week of hospitalization. Crysdale's (1989) reported results were 20% excellent, 47% good, 22% fair, and 11% poor, with 194 patients with at least 1-year follow-up. Eight percent of the patients developed ranulas, which are cystic accumulations of saliva in the floor of the mouth arising from the sublingual glands. He now recommends simultaneous sublingual gland excision. Two percent of the patients required submandibular gland excision because of obstruction or cyst formation.

The author of this chapter transposes the ducts to the base of the tongue and has never felt tonsillectomy was necessary (see Figures 10.1 to 10.4). Tonsillectomy and adenoidectomy may, however, be indicated for nasopharyngeal obstruction that causes mouth breathing. Saliva control may improve in a patient who has corrected airway obstruction. During the procedure, meticulous technique is used to minimize trauma to the submandibular ducts, and during the transposition, special care is taken to avoid kinking of the ducts that may cause obstruction.

Hotaling, Madgy, Kuhns, Filipek, and Belenky (1992) reported the results of radioneucleotide studies following submandibular duct transposition. They found that 2 of 12 submandibular glands ceased to function, indicating that trauma to the duct or kinking led to, what was in effect, duct ligation. Crysdale et al. (2001) showed no function in 10 of 22 glands similarly studied. This supports the new concept (Klem & Mair, 1999) that submandibular duct ligation may be efficacious and safe in severely disabled patients such as those who are tube fed but suffer breathing difficulties due to excessive production of saliva, which cannot effectively be swallowed. These patients would otherwise be candidates for tracheostomy.

Sublingual Gland Excision

This surgery is done through the same anterior floor of mouth incision as for submandibular duct transposition (see Figures 10.1 to 10.4). It requires careful dissection of the duct and lingual nerve branches, protecting the terminal hypoglossal nerve. Strict hemostasis of large sublingual arteries and veins is essential, which adds 30 minutes to duct rerouting. A large tributary from the sublingual glands entering the submandibular duct is frequently found, and this must be divided prior to duct rerouting. Presumably there would be a high risk of ranula formation in these cases if the sublingual tissue drained by this accessory duct went on to accumulate saliva. The addition of sublingual gland excision to submandibular duct transposition was first suggested by Crysdale (1992).

THE MELBOURNE EXPERIENCE

Up until 1993, at the Royal Children's Hospital (RCH) in Melbourne, the standard technique used for salivary control surgery consisted of bilateral submandibular duct transposition and unilateral parotid duct ligation. C. Bennett (personal communication, 1990)

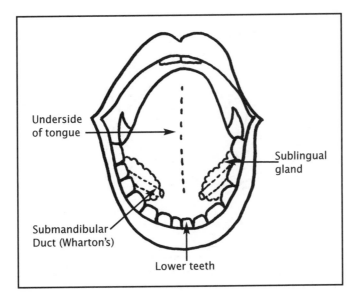

FIGURE 10.1. The relationship of the submandibular ducts to the sublingual glands and the lingual nerves below the mucosa of the floor of the mouth.

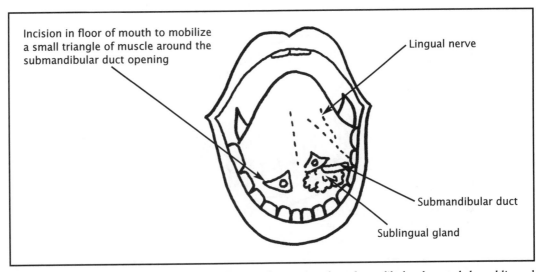

FIGURE 10.2. Incisions in the floor of the mouth exposing the submandibular duct and the sublingual gland on the patient's left side.

reported that in 65 patients, 30% were much better, 50% were significantly improved, and 20% were not improved. No patient was made worse, but there was a tendency for some patients to relapse over 6 to 12 months. Some patients have had thick stringy saliva and mucus deposits on the lips. Five percent of the patients developed ranulas.

A 5- to 8-year follow-up of some RCH patients using a variety of measures has been reported (Webb, Reddihough, Johnson, Bennett, & Byrt, 1995). All 28 patients measured pre- and post-operatively using the drooling quotient improved; the median quotients being 50.0 preoperatively and 12.3 postoperatively ($p < .001$). The severity of drooling decreased in 28 of 36 patients (78%) and the frequency decreased in 32 of 35 patients (91%). Both the median severity and frequency scores improved by 1.3 grades. A caregiver's review by questionnaire, however, revealed that only 24 of 39 (61%) found the surgery helpful. Two patients (5%) had postoperative airway obstruction and 5 patients

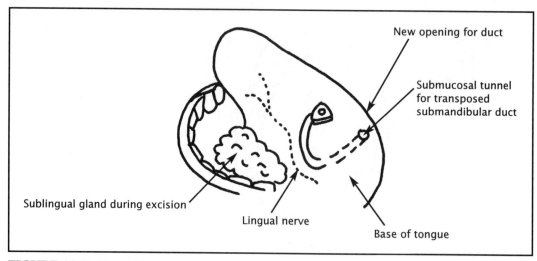

FIGURE 10.3. View of the tongue and the floor of the mouth from the left side showing mobilization of the submandibular duct prior to relocation and sublingual gland excision.

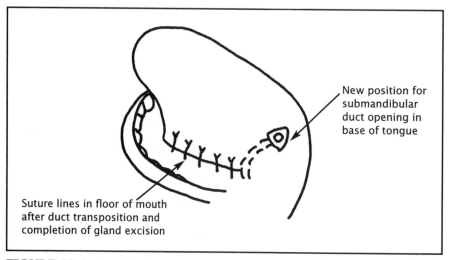

FIGURE 10.4. Completed surgery.

(13%) developed ranulas. Five patients had an increase in dental caries anecdotally, 9 reported a dry mouth with crusting, and 18 (46%) described their saliva as thicker, with 6 reporting more difficulty swallowing.

Excessive dental decay, particularly involving the lower central teeth, has been reported (Hallett, Lucas, Johnston, Reddihough, & Hall, 1995). These patients mostly had bilateral submandibular duct transposition with or without unilateral parotid duct ligation. Anecdotally, some cases show more marked dental caries on the side of parotid duct ligation.

Since 1993, the author of this chapter followed Crysdale's lead and added bilateral sublingual gland excision to bilateral submandibular duct transposition. This excision has eliminated ranula formation and may improve the control of sialorrhea, possibly without need for parotid duct ligation. It also is felt that this may prevent the development of thick tenacious saliva, seen when only the submandibular ducts are transposed with a single parotid duct ligation. If the initial operation has not produced a satisfactory outcome, it is possible to add a unilateral parotid duct ligation as a secondary procedure.

The chapter author's personal series consists of 70 bilateral submandibular duct transpositions with bilateral sublingual gland excision. Five of these patients who had unsatisfactory outcomes went on to have an additional parotid duct ligation. The extent of dental caries has decreased during this period, although improved oral hygiene and dental surveillance have been instituted. Details of prophylactic dental strategies can be found in Chapter 4.

Bilateral parotid duct ligations were carried out in 2 patients who have previous failed bilateral submandibular duct transpositions and in 2 patients with Moebius syndrome, with tracheostomies. One patient had a tongue reduction. In those patients undergoing bilateral submandibular duct transposition and bilateral sublingual gland excision, complications were minor in 5 patients (7%) and major in 4 patients (6%). These complications include bleeding, which was minor in 1 child and major in 2. One patient who had major bleeding problems was found to have high sodium velproate levels, which are known to affect platelets. Tongue swelling causing airway obstruction was short lived in 2 children and prolonged in 1 child. There was 1 patient with a submandibular abscess, 1 with lingual nerve division, and 1 with aspiration pneumonia. In 9 patients (13%), anatomical anomalies or difficult access to the mouth made surgery challenging.

Of the 70 patients who have had bilateral submandibular duct transpositions with bilateral sublingual gland excision, 49 have been studied prospectively. Postoperative follow-up consists of review at 1, 6, and 12 months and at 2 and 5 years. The rating scales and questionnaires used are found in Appendix A.

Table 10.1 shows the diagnoses that have been assigned to the 49 patients. Of these patients, 22 have an additional diagnosis of epilepsy. Prospective review has identified 5 more patients who had postoperative difficulties, such as delayed resumption of feeding, pain, and a seizure. A complete data set for all prospectively followed patients is not yet available. A summary of results to date follows:

- Drooling frequency: Of 46 patients, 31 (67.4%) had an improved score (see Table 10.2). The mean frequency score fell 0.87 points from 3.6 to 2.7 within 2 years of follow-up ($p < .0001$).

- Drooling severity: Of 46 patients, 37 (80.4%) had an improved score (see Table 10.3). The mean severity score fell 1.4 points from 4.5 to 3.0 within 2 years of follow-up ($p < .0001$).

TABLE 10.1
Diagnoses of Children Who Had Surgery, 1993–2001

Diagnosis	Number of Patients
Cerebral palsy	28
Intellectual disability	15
Developmental delay	4
Other	2
Total	**49**

TABLE 10.2

Drooling Frequency Changes from Presurgery to Postsurgery

Change in Frequency Score	Number of Patients	Percentage of Patients
-1 (worse)	4	8.70
0 (no change)	11	23.91
1 (better)	21	45.65
2	7	15.22
3	3	6.52
Total	**46**	**100.00**

TABLE 10.3

Drooling Severity Changes from Presurgery to Postsurgery

Change in Severity Score (pre–post surgery)	Number of Patients	Percentage of Patients
-1 (worse)	3	6.52
0 (no change)	6	13.04
1 (better)	15	32.61
2	14	30.43
3	7	15.22
4	1	2.17
Total	**46**	**100.00**

- Changes of clothes or bibs per day: Data on this item are available on 29 patients, of whom 24 (82.8%) reported improvement after 2 years with a mean fall of 3.35 from 4.2 to 0.86 ($p < .0001$). The numbers of bibs changed per day ranged from 1 to 14 preoperatively and ranged from 0 to 5 postoperatively.

- "Reduction in drooling" as assessed as a percentage by caregivers showed a median reduction of 60% at 2 years. The data available on 39 patients is not normally distributed. The Wilcoxon signed rank test indicated a level of statistical significance of $p < .0001$. Only 3 patients (8%) were assessed by caregivers as not improving, and 72% of caregivers reported 50% or more reduction in drooling.

- Changes in saliva consistency were noted in 27 patients. When given a choice of clear, opaque, or frothy, 14 (52%) said it was still clear, 7 (26%) said it was opaque, and 6 (22%) had frothy saliva. When asked to rate their saliva as watery, slightly sticky, or thick or mucousy, 12 (44%) rated their saliva as watery, 11 (41%) as slightly sticky, and 4 (15%) as mucousy. When asked about the odor of the saliva, 12 (25%) reported the smell of their saliva to be offensive.

Preliminary data supports the view that about 4 out of 5 patients benefit from surgery, with half showing a marked improvement (i.e., 2 or more points improvement on the severity scale) and 72% of caregivers report 50% or more reduction in drooling. The number of bibs used or clothes changed per day decreased from more than four preoperatively to less than one on average. Six percent of patients experience a major complication.

 CASE STUDY

In 1994, a 7-year-old girl underwent bilateral submandibular duct transposition and sublingual gland excision for uncontrolled sialorrhea. She needed up to 12 bibs changed per day. A trial of benzhexol was unsuccessful because of the side effect of nightmares. Her diagnosis was that of quadraparetic cerebral palsy, associated with moderate developmental delay. She came from a rural community where the water was not flurodated. In 1992, she had a number of dental extractions and restorations under general anesthesia for dental decay.

The surgery was uncomplicated, with the return to oral fluids and a soft diet after 2 days. She was discharged on the third postoperative day. Her sialorrhea slowly decreased over a 3-month period, and since that time she has worn no bibs nor required changes of clothes. She has had further dental restorations in 1996 and 2000. Orthopedically she has required multilevel lower limb surgery following gait analysis and has had botulinum toxin injection into her more spastic right upper limb. Dental decay continues to be a problem and this now includes her lower central incisors, which are usually spared.

Review at the age of 14 years reveals that she is progressing well at school, although there is still some drooling, which is described as "stringy." This drool wets her schoolwork, stains her clothes, and produces an unpleasant odor. She is well accepted by her peers but does have some cosmetic concerns about her drooling. A further trial of benzhexol has been unsuccessful, once again due to nightmares, but a new trial of glycopyrrolate, which has fewer central nervous system effects, has been instituted.

REFERENCES

Chaushu, G., Dori, S., Sela, B. A., Taicher, S., Kronenberg, J., & Talmi, Y. P. (2001). Salivary flow dynamics after parotid surgery: A preliminary report. *Otolaryngology—Head and Neck Surgery, 124*(3), 270–273.

Crysdale, W. S. (1980). The drooling patient: Evaluation and current surgical options. *Laryngoscope, 90,* 775–783.

Crysdale, W. S. (1989). Management options for the drooling patient. *Ear, Nose, and Throat Journal, 68*(11), 820–830.

Crysdale, W. S. (1992). Drooling: Experience with team assessment and management. *Clinical Pediatrics, 31*(2), 77–80.

Crysdale, W. S., Raveh, E., McCann, C., Roskee, L., & Aiona, M. (2001). Management of drooling in individuals with neurodisability: A surgical experience. *Developmental Medicine and Child Neurology, 43*(6), 379–383.

Dundas, D. F., & Peterson, R. A. (1979). Surgical treatment of drooling by bilateral parotid duct ligation and submandibular gland resection. *Plastic Reconstructive Surgery, 64*(1), 47–51.

Hallett, K. B., Lucas, J. O., Johnston, T., Reddihough, D. S., & Hall, R. K. (1995). Dental health of children with cerebral palsy following sialodochoplasty. *Special Care in Dentistry, 15*(6), 234–238.

Hotaling, A. J., Madgy, D. N., Kuhns, L. R., Filipek, L., & Belenky, W. M. (1992). Postoperative technetium scanning in patients with submandibular duct diversion. *Archives of Otolaryngology—Head and Neck Surgery, 118*(12), 1331–1333.

Klem, C., & Mair, E. A. (1999). Four-duct ligation: A simple and effective treatment for chronic aspiration from sialorrhea. *Archives of Otolaryngology—Head and Neck Surgery, 125*(7), 796–800.

Varma, S. K., Henderson, H. P., & Cotton, B. R. (1991). Treatment of drooling by parotid duct ligation and submandibular diversion. *British Journal of Plastic Surgery, 44,* 415–417.

Webb, K., Reddihough, D. S., Johnson, H., Bennett, C. S., & Byrt, T. (1995). Long-term outcome of saliva-control surgery. *Developmental Medicine and Child Neurology, 37*(9), 755–762.

Wilkie, T. F. (1967). The problem of drooling in cerebral palsy: A surgical approach. *Canadian Journal of Surgery, 10,* 60–67.

Wilkie, T. F., & Brody, G. S. (1977). The surgical treatment of drooling: A ten year review. *Journal of Plastic and Reconstructive Surgery, 59*(6), 791–798.

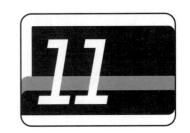

Complementary Strategies for Drooling and Xerostomia

Learning Outcomes

- *Have an understanding of a range of complementary strategies used in the management of drooling*

- *Gain an overview of a range of complementary strategies used in the management of xerostomia*

- *Be aware that these approaches lack empirical evidence and require careful monitoring of outcomes*

- *Understand the need to trial different approaches in consultation with the clients, caregivers, or both*

Many people choose to deal with their saliva problems by using nonmedical means. Sometimes, even after all possible interventions, a drooling problem will remain and clinicians and clients may wish to use a complementary approach. In this chapter, we deal with feedback from people with the problem and how they have dealt with it.

In Chapter 2, we talked about a team approach and how complementary medicine may have a role in saliva control. Some examples of this follow.

POINT PERCUSSION THERAPY

Point percussion is a type of acupressure therapy, Dian Xue, which is popular in Melbourne, Australia. It includes massaging and triggering specific points. It has its roots in Eastern medicine, and the major practitioners originate from China. A number of parents have reported success in reducing drooling in their children with cerebral palsy.

Treatment for drooling consists of applying point percussion therapy for approximately 10 minutes daily, 5 days a week. The length of treatment varies from 2 weeks for mild drooling to 4 weeks for more severe difficulties. Change should be noticeable in 2 weeks.

The practitioner demonstrates the procedure to the parent or caregiver when the patient is lying in the supine position. The pressure on the points can cause discomfort for the child, and it is suggested that you use as much pressure as the person can bear. The parent or caregiver is taught to administer the treatment so that it can be continued on a regular basis. Parents have reported that although the treatment can be effective for drooling, it is not long term. However, when the drooling returns they then need to repeat the treatment.

A short study was conducted with three adults with cerebral palsy. Therapists were trained in the technique. One adult improved, but this was very short term. Another person found it too painful.

ACUPUNCTURE

Although acupuncture is now widely accepted as being helpful for many medical conditions, there is very little literature reporting on efficacy for drooling. One study (Wong, Sun, & Wong, 2001) applied tongue acupuncture to 10 children for 30 sessions over 6 weeks. The children had severe disabilities and epilepsy and were unable to cognitively follow directions. Tongue acupuncture was applied to five points on the tongue using an acupuncture needle while the child was sitting on the mother's knee. It was reported that all children tolerated the treatment well and that their drooling decreased by the completion of the study. There was no control group in the study, nor any long-term outcomes.

It may be that Eastern medicine has some approaches to drooling that we could use. Both approaches mentioned that there was some pain involved, and this may or may not be acceptable to some individuals.

HERBAL MEDICATIONS

Several commercially available herbal products have been used to reduce the amount of saliva. The most frequently used products are horseradish tablets and astringent teas, such as hibiscus and sage tea. Again, the efficacy of these products has not been assessed; however, some people report that they are useful.

CLOTHING AND CLOTHING PROTECTORS

Clothing can be adapted to minimize dampness and conceal visual signs of drooling (Chambers & Franklin, 1992). A very young child can wear a bib to mop up the excess saliva, but this becomes inappropriate as the child grows older. Consider some general principles when choosing clothing.

Clothing should be selected to do the following:

- It should be absorbent. The level of absorbency is dependent on the fibers. Cotton or cotton viscose mixture with a high percentage of cotton is absorbent. The most absorbent fabrics are knitted or textured (e.g., seersucker or waffle) or have a brushed looped or pile finish.

- Clothing should minimize the physical discomfort of dampness against the skin and protect the skin. The ideal waterproof backing is washable, lightweight, noiseless, and microporous, such as those used in good quality rainwear.

- It should be removable without being pulled over the head.

- It should have no fastenings in areas that are likely to get wet. Snaps are better than zippers if they get wet.

- Clothing should disguise wet areas and distract attention from them. Patterned fabric with an irregular multicolored design or with light and dark shades of the same color disguise wet patches better than plain fabrics do.

The following are other ideas and adaptions you might try:

- Use removable items such as scarves, cravats, bows, and collars to wear around the neck. (You may need a variety of these items in different colors to match various outfits.)

- Wear toweling panels for sweatshirts. These sweatshirts can be attached with hook-and-loop fasteners (see Figure 11.1).

- Choose sweatshirts with raised motifs (the sweatshirt appears dryer for longer).

- Try terry cloth tops gathered into a roll neck that fits snugly around the neck.

- Sew velcro onto spandex sleeves, which can slip around a seat belt and form a cover, to protect a harness or belt from getting wet. They are easily changed.

- Try putting sweatbands on the child's wrist if the child can wipe his or her chin. The chin can be wiped with the wrist rather than the child having to carry a handkerchief.

- Sew an absorbent paper sheet (such as those used as incontinence aids) onto a towel that is worn like a toweling top (see Figure 11.2). The sheet absorbs the moisture and does not irritate the skin.

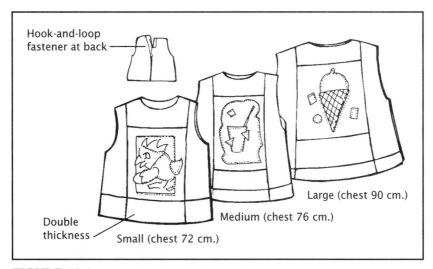

FIGURE 11.1. Sweatshirts for absorbing saliva.

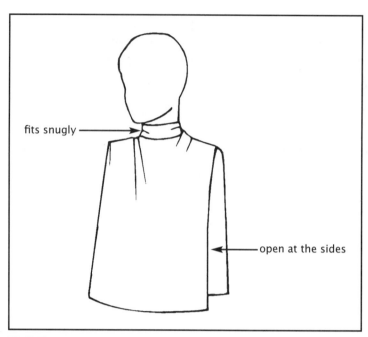

FIGURE 11.2. Toweling tops for saliva protection.

DISGUISING THE ODOR

When stale saliva makes clothing smell, try a drop of an essential oil, such as eucalyptus or lavender, cologne, or deodorizer on the clothes. There are many commercially available odor eaters.

ENVIRONMENTAL PROPS

- Raise the work or school space (by using a slant-board desk, for instance) so that the person does not have to spend long periods with the head down.

- If the person is in a wheelchair, angle the back of the chair so that the person's head and neck are tipped back and the head and body are at the same angle in a straight line, slightly backward.

- If the person is hospitalized or in a wheelchair, a gooseneck rod can be attached to the head of the bed or to the wheelchair, with a foam ball on the end. The person can use the foam ball for wiping.

STRATEGIES FOR XEROSTOMIA OR STICKY SALIVA

Acupuncture also has been used to assist with xerostomia (Blom, Dawidson, & Angmar-Mänsson, 1992). Twenty-one adults with severe xerostomia were randomly assigned to a placebo or acupuncture group. Acupuncture and placebo acupuncture were given twice a week for 20 minutes for two 6-week periods. Measurements were taken at baseline, 7, 16, 28, 40, and 64 weeks. All patients who received the treatment improved their saliva flow, with 4 patients attaining normal salivary flow rates. The improvements lasted during the year of observation. Some of the placebo group also showed improvement in flow, but this was transitory, ceasing when the treatment ceased.

MAINTAINING ORAL HEALTH

Xerostomia results in the loss of the natural barrier that protects the mucous membranes. A severe reduction of saliva leads to the loss of the protective antiseptic properties, the contribution to clearing material from the mouth, and the buffering effects against acidity.

Saliva also has an important role in eating and drinking. Saliva lubricates the food and makes it easier to swallow and it mediates taste and smell. After meals, there is an increase in the amount of saliva secreted. This saliva helps move the food through the esophagus and into the stomach, and it reduces the likelihood of reflux.

Many people with oral dryness experience oral infections, such as thrush (*Candida albincans*). The resultant mouth discomfort and painful swallowing may lead people to avoid eating. The following oral health plan is aimed at preventing problems associated with oral dryness and infections and treating them promptly when they occur. There are two components of this program: prevention and treatment.

Prevention

- Keep the mouth clean and moist.

- Increase water intake. Carry a water bottle and sip it regularly or suck ice chips. The aim is to have a liter of plain water every day.

- Always rinse the mouth with plain water after eating and drinking. Rinsing is particularly important if a person has a dry mouth because residual food particles may irritate the gums.

- Brush with a soft bristle toothbrush, because this avoids scraping the gums.

- Use dental floss at least once a day to remove debris that may lead to irritation or infections.

- Use a lip moisturizer to prevent cracking and dryness.

- Use an oral lubricant, either commercially available artificial saliva, or a vegetable oil that coats the mouth with a film to help protect the mucous membranes.

- Chew sugarless gum. The act of chewing stimulates saliva production.

- Teas, such as lemon tea, can increase the amount of saliva produced. However, some teas (for example, hibiscus and rose hip) actually seem to leave the mouth feeling drier.

- When troubled by thick tenacious saliva the use of mucolitic enzymes, such as papain, which is extracted from the papaya, can be helpful. They can be obtained in tablet form from the health food shop. These tablets can be useful when sucked, because they break down the proteins in the saliva and make the saliva thinner and easier to swallow.

- Fruit acids have mucolitic properties; people have reported that fruit juices, such as dark grape juice, thins down the thick saliva in their mouth.

Avoid things that may cause or exacerbate oral problems:

- Commercial mouthwashes often contain alcohol, hydrogen peroxide, or both. These ingredients have a drying effect on the mouth.

- Sucking candies and other foods that are high in sugar can worsen a fungal infection and lead to dental caries.

Treatment

- Treat any oral sores or infections as soon as they occur and follow advice given.

- Sometimes people with low-grade chronic oral infections ignore problems until they are severe and more difficult to treat.

- Rinse a sore mouth in a solution of ½ teaspoon of bicarbonate soda in 1 cup of water at least four times per day and after meals.

- Have a moist soft diet and add sauces and gravies because they are less likely to make the mouth sore or scrape the mucous membranes.

- Avoid serving food that is very hot and could irritate the mouth.

- Avoid fizzy drinks that can irritate mouth sores and cause a burning sensation.

- Avoid alcoholic drinks and cigarettes.

- Eat foods that are nutrient dense. This includes food supplements such as Ensure. If there are any problems eating an adequate amount of food, contact a dietitian for advice. It is a good idea to follow a milk-based supplement with a small amount of fruit juice or water to wash through any residue, because milk-based products have been reported to increase the viscosity of the saliva (Enderby, 1995).

To date, there has been little empirical research as to the efficacy of the management strategies described in this chapter. There is a need to develop the evidence for these interventions. However, these strategies have been applied clinically, with clients reporting that they are beneficial. Clinicians should adopt a collaborative approach with clients and related professionals to experiment and try to find the compensatory strategies that most effectively address the specific problems of the person.

REFERENCES

Blom, M., Dawidson, I., & Angmar-Mänsson, B. (1992, March). The effect of acupuncture on salivary flow rates in patients with xerostomia. *Oral Surgery, Oral Medicine, Oral Pathology*, 293–298.

Chambers, D., & Franklin, L. (1992). *Creative clothing—Practical options for people who have difficulty with saliva control*. West Perth, Australia: Western Australian Association of Occupational Therapists.

Enderby, P. C. E. (1995). The effect of dairy products on the viscosity of saliva. *Clinical Rehabilitation, 9*(1), 61–64.

Wong, V., Sun, J. G., & Wong, W. (2001). Traditional Chinese medicine (tongue acupuncture) in children with drooling problems. *Pediatric Neurology, 25*, 47–54.

APPENDIX

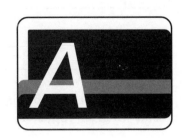

Assessment Forms

- *Saliva Control Assessment*
- *Drooling Rating Scale*
- *Post–Saliva-Surgery Form*
- *Oral Secretion Assessment*

Saliva Control Assessment

Date _____

Name _____ Date of Birth _____

Please answer the following questions about your child with a yes or no and write additional comments when appropriate.

1. Communication Skills

    _____ No problem

    _____ Some speech

    _____ Uses speech to get message across but with difficulty

    _____ Has difficulty making some sounds in words

    _____ Has no speech

2. Walking

    _____ No difficulty

    _____ Needs a walking aid

    _____ Uses a wheelchair

3. Head Position

    _____ Can hold head up with difficulty

    _____ Tends to sit with head down mostly

4. Mouth

    _____ Is the mouth always open?

5. Lips

    _____ Can hold lips together easily and for a long time

    _____ Can hold lips together for a limited time

    _____ Can hold lips together with effort for a limited time

    _____ Can bring lips together only briefly

    _____ Unable to bring lips together

    _____ Can pucker lips (as in a kiss)

6. Tongue

    _____ Pushes tongue out when swallowing

7. Straw

    _____ Can use a straw easily

    _____ Has difficulty using a straw

    _____ Cannot use a straw

8. Eating

_____ Can eat whole foods and hard foods that are difficult to eat

_____ Needs to have food cut into small pieces

_____ Foods need to be mashed

_____ Foods need to be pureed

_____ Has food through a tube (nasogastric/gastrostomy)

_____ Can eat independently but is a messy eater

9. Swallowing

_____ Can he or she swallow on demand?

10. Sensation

_____ Does he or she notice the saliva on lips or chin (perhaps tries to wipe chin)?

11. Does he or she need to change clothes or wear bibs because of excess saliva?

_____ If yes, how many times a day? _____

12. Does the saliva cause an unpleasant odor? _____

13. Good General Health

_____ Has asthma

_____ Has frequently blocked or runny nose

_____ Has bouts of pneumonia

14. Dental Care

_____ Does he or she see a dentist?

_____ Any problems with bleeding gums or decayed teeth?

15. Does he or she sometimes have dry days with no drooling?

_____ If yes, are these more frequent than they used to be? _____

When Is Drooling Worst?	N/A	Yes	No	DK
When tired				
When has a cold				
When concentrating on a task				
When watching TV				
When head is down				
When excited, angry, upset				
When talking				
When eating or drinking				
After eating or drinking				
When hands or objects in mouth				

When Is Drooling Worst?	N/A	Yes	No	DK
Before seizures				
After seizures				
When in pain				
When bored				
When asleep				
When teething, or has sore mouth				
When writing, drawing, or making things with hands				

Note. N/A = not applicable; DK = don't know.

16. Does he or she have epilepsy?

_____ If yes, please include names and doses of any medications

_____

_____

17. Is he or she on any other medication?

_____ If yes, please include the names and dosage

_____

_____

Please circle the number that best answers the following questions:

18. How much of a problem is drooling?

0------------1------------2------------3------------4------------5

19. To what extent does the individual's drooling affect his or her life?

0------------1------------2------------3------------4------------5

20. To what extent does the individual's drooling affect you and your family's life?

0------------1------------2------------3------------4------------5

Please add any comments:

_____

_____

_____

_____

_____

_____

_____

Thank you for taking the time to answer these questions.

Drooling Rating Scale

The accurate measurement of drooling is difficult because it can vary from day to day and activity to activity. We use rating scales to assess the severity and frequency of drooling.

This scale has two parts: Frequency and Severity.

Frequency

1   No drooling—dry

2   Occasional drooling (not every day)

3   Frequent drooling (every day but not all the time)

4   Constant drooling—always wet

Severity

1   Dry—never drools

2   Mild—only the lips are wet

3   Moderate—wet on the lips and the chin

4   Severe—drools to the extent that clothes get damp and need changing

5   Profuse—clothing, hands, and objects become wet

Please discuss these items with anyone who knows the individual well, and work out which numbers best reflect the frequency and severity of drooling. If possible, it is useful if this form can be completed every day for 5 days. It also is helpful if two people from different environments can complete the form (e.g., home and school).

To Use the Scale

1. It is preferable that two sets of people should complete the scale daily. The scales should be scored separately and not involve discussion between the two scorers, for example, a teacher at school and a parent at home.

2. It is advisable to complete the scale at the end of the day. Rating should be for 5 to 10 days. Longer measures (10 days) are particularly useful if the individual's drooling varies from day to day.

3. On the enclosed chart, record the number that corresponds to the frequency and severity of drooling (see Rating Scale Chart). Each rater needs his or her own chart on which to record the rating number.

Rating Scale Chart

Name of individual being rated _____

Date of Observation	Frequency	Severity	Initials of Rater	Comments

Post–Saliva-Surgery Form

Name of individual _____

Date _____ Date of surgery _____ Number of bib changes a day _____

Number of clothing changes a day _____

How much do you think the drooling has reduced since the operation (e.g., 20%, 100%)? _____

Please check the answer (just one on each line) that best answers the following questions:

1. Is the quality of the saliva the same as before the surgery?

    ☐ Yes   ☐ No

    If no, choose all items from the following that describe the saliva:

    ☐ Clear   ☐ Opaque   ☐ Frothy
    ☐ Watery   ☐ Slightly sticky   ☐ Thick or mucousy
    ☐ No odor   ☐ Sometimes offensive   ☐ Offensive odor
    ☐ Does not leave the chin ☐ Falls in strings   ☐ Falls in drops
    ☐ Easily wiped   ☐ Requires firm wipe   ☐ Needs persistent wipe
    ☐ Normal lips   ☐ Moist lips   ☐ Crusty lips

2. Has the individual's medication changed since the operation?

    ☐ Yes   ☐ No

    If yes, please explain: _____

    _____

    _____

3. To what extent does the individual's drooling affect his or her life?

         0------------1------------2------------3------------4------------5
    Not at all   Greatly

    Comments: _____

    _____

    _____

4. To what extent does the individual's drooling affect you or your family's life?

         0------------1------------2------------3------------4------------5
    Not at all   Greatly

    Comments: _____

    _____

    _____

5. How much of a problem is the individual's drooling?

0------------1------------2------------3------------4------------5

Not at all   Serious problem

Comments: _____

_____

_____

6. When is the drooling at its worst?

When Is Drooling Worst?	N/A	Yes	No	DK
When tired				
When has a cold				
When concentrating on a task				
When watching TV				
When head is down				
When excited, angry, upset				
When talking				
When eating or drinking				
After eating or drinking				
When hands or objects in mouth				
Before seizures				
After seizures				
When in pain				
When bored				
When asleep				
When teething or has sore mouth				
When writing, drawing, or making things with hands				

Note. N/A = not applicable; DK = don't know.

7. Any other comments? _____

_____

_____

_____

_____

_____

_____

Oral Secretion Assessment

Name _____ Date _____

Date	Breakfast		Midmorning		Lunch		Midafternoon		Dinner		Evening	
	Before	After	Before	After	Before	After	Before	After	Before	After	Before	After

Instructions

1. Evaluate your oral secretions before and after eating or drinking for each day. If you do not eat or drink anything at any time of the assessment time, simply fill in the "before" space for that time.

2. Fill in the form on 3 days for 1 week (the days do not have to be consecutive).

3. Use the symbols listed below and add the plus signs if they more accurately describe the nature of your oral secretions.

Key to Rating System

N = Normal—mouth or pharynx coated with saliva (1)

D = Dry—mouth dry or uncomfortable (2)

R = Ropy or thick secretions (2)

W = Aware of watery saliva (2)

Qualifications

+ = Excessive

++ = Very excessive

APPENDIX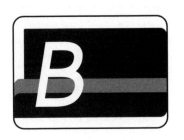

Caregiver Training Materials

- *Getting That Tongue Going*
- *Using a Full Intraoral Appliance Such as an ISMAR*
- *Helping Your Child To Feel the Saliva*
- *Helping Your Child Toward a Dry Chin*
- *Getting Those Lips Together and Working*
- *Keeping Up Appearances*

Getting That Tongue Going

Sometimes the child's tongue does not have the flexibility or speed of movement to eat neatly or speak clearly. Here are some ideas to help the tongue move more.

- Put chips of ice in the child's mouth, especially before eating.
- Use a thin icy pole made from frozen water:
  1. Stroke from the ear to the corner of the lips three times on both sides. At the end of this stroking encourage the child to swallow.
  2. Stroke around the mouth. Go from the middle of the lip to the edge on both upper and lower lips. Do each quadrant three times. Encourage the child to close lips together and swallow.
- Freeze cotton swabs and run them down the center of the child's tongue (in the groove) front to back. Allow the child to swallow in between.
- Usually the child's tongue will move toward where you are touching in the mouth. If this happens you can play games with the tongue.

Games To Play with the Tongue:

- move the tongue in and out like a lizard's,
- do big slow movements like licking a plate,
- waggle the tongue from side to side like a snake's,
- lick the lips like a crocodile after his last meal,
- click the tongue,
- pretend to be a cat licking its paws,
- look in the mirror and push the tongue against the cheeks, and
- put different tastes and textures in the mouth to help the tongue to move around. Try things like peanut butter and flavored spreads. Put a little bit on the top lip, on the bottom lip, and at the side of the mouth. Place the textures so the child needs to use the tongue to get to the "reward."

Using a Full Intraoral Appliance Such as an ISMAR

ISMARs (Innsbruck Sensori Motor Activator and Regulator) are designed to provide stability for the jaw to develop lip and tongue ability. There are a number of different designs (see Figure B.1). For children with good steady jaws, you might only use an upper plate. The plates are designed to fit in the mouth and encourage the lips and tongue to move using different movements. The design of the plates needs the assistance of a dentist and a speech–language pathologist. Your child needs to be able to tolerate having an impression taken and also the putting in and taking out of the appliance. Your child needs to be able to breathe through his or her nose. Every few weeks, the plates are altered; for example, grooves are put into the plate or beads are attached. These changes make the plate feel different and then your child's tongue is encouraged to explore the inside of the mouth more. The ISMAR is only used for short periods of time, about 2 to 3 minutes, building up to 30 minutes. Once this is achieved, it can then be worn overnight as passive therapy. The devices are worn for a few weeks or up to 5 years depending on your child's goals and abilities.

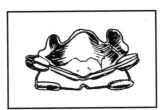

FIGURE B.1. Innsbruck Sensori Motor Activator and Regulator (ISMAR).

Helping Your Child To Feel the Saliva

Many children do not seem to notice the saliva until it is too late. When we get enough saliva in our mouths we swallow it automatically, thus we do not dribble. This does not seem to happen to children who dribble. Some children seem very unaware of what is in and around their mouths, and they can be messy eaters.

Here are some strategies to help. Please be guided by your speech–language pathologist as to which strategies are most appropriate.

OUTSIDE OF THE MOUTH

Vibration

Battery-operated vibrators can be used to stimulate the muscles in the cheeks and around the lips. Vibrators come in all sorts of shapes (see Figures B.2 through B.6), but use a small one (or one with a small head).[1] You also can use the back of the head of a battery-operated toothbrush (e.g., Reach powerbrush).

1. Vibrate from the ear to the corner of the lips three times on both sides, then encourage the child to swallow.

2. Vibrate around the mouth. Go from the middle of the lip to the edge on both upper and lower lips. Do each quadrant three times. Encourage the child to close the lips together and swallow.

You can make this into a game, for example, shaving.

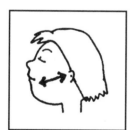

FIGURE B.2. Face with arrows (side).

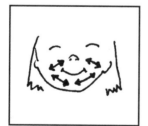

FIGURE B.3. Face with arrows (front).

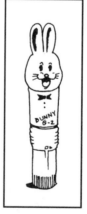

FIGURE B.4. Bunny vibrator.

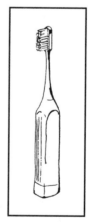

FIGURE B.5. Toothbrush.

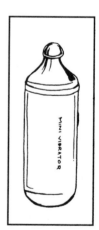

FIGURE B.6. Minivibrator.

---

[1] You can buy vibrators from a number of different sources. The big body massagers are too big for children. One example of a massager designed for oral–facial stimulation is the Jiggler Fun Facial and Oral Massager from Abilitations (phone: 800/850-8602; fax: 800/845-1535; e-mail: orders@sportime.com; Web: www.abilitations.com).

INSIDE THE MOUTH

Icing

The use of ice can heighten a dull sensation. The research has shown that touching the fauces (arches at the back of the mouth) with a thin stick of ice has increased the ability to swallow frequently. This is very difficult to do with children; however, you can try.

1. Put chips of ice in the child's mouth, especially before eating.

2. Use ice in the same way as described in the Vibration section. Use a thin icy pole made from frozen water.

3. Freeze cotton swabs and run them down the center of the child's tongue (in the groove) front to back. Allow the child to swallow in between.

Very young children or children who are very sensitive in the mouth may need help to tolerate anything in their mouths. Usually we try with fingers (ours and theirs) exploring the mouth, using a firm touch on their gums. We also can use toys and different foods. Some of the toys that are useful are animal rubber toys, because they are easy to clean and have a range of shapes (see Figure B.7).

Using Taste and Texture

Different tastes and textures in the mouth can help the tongue to move around in the mouth. Try things like vegemite (a salty savory spread), peanut butter, hundreds and thousands (small multi-colored sugar balls), flavored spreads. Put a little bit up under the top lip, outside and inside the teeth, behind the bottom lip, just behind the top teeth, and between the cheek and the lower teeth. Place the textures so the child needs to use the tongue or lips to get to the "reward."

Toothbrushing

1. The use of an electric toothbrush used three times a day is very good for the gums and the teeth.

2. If the toothbrush is too strong, use a gentle finger toothbrush (infadents; see Figure B.8) and rub the gums three times on each side from front to back. Do this before a meal.

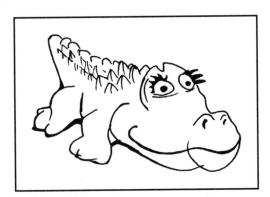

FIGURE B.7. Alligator chew toy.

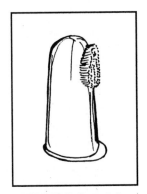

FIGURE B.8. Infadent.

Helping Your Child Toward a Dry Chin

Lots of children who dribble have difficulty knowing if their lips and chin are wet, thus they do not think to wipe. We can often help with this by putting in place ways and methods to help children remember to do this. We need the following:

1. something to wipe with,
2. a cue to wipe, and
3. a reward for wiping.

SOMETHING TO WIPE WITH

Many children find getting a hankie out of a pocket a difficult thing to do. For those children, it may be possible for them to wear a sweatband on the wrist for them to wipe their chin. Some children have a hankie tied to their wrists for easy access. Some people who are in wheelchairs have a foam ball on a gooseneck stand. A hankie is placed over the ball and changed at the appropriate interval.

A CUE FOR WIPING

If your child does not notice the saliva coming out of his or her mouth, he or she needs a cue for wiping. It also can be useful to teach "swallow and wipe" together, because then the mouth is cleared of saliva each time you wipe. At first you might have to remind your child to wipe, and this needs to be very frequent. Soon you will feel like a broken record and need to find some other way. The following suggestions may be useful:

- Use touch cues. Sometimes pressing the flat of your finger on your child's top lip helps him or her to swallow. Touching your child's chin or lip also may be a touch cue.

- Use visual cues, for example, colored dots, so when your child sees these cues a swallow or wipe occurs. Or you can touch your lips with your finger as a cue.

- Use auditory cues; for example, set an oven timer and encourage your child to swallow or wipe after the buzzer, use a buzzer that goes into an earplug in your child's ear,[1] or read a book and swallow and wipe every two pages.

REWARD FOR WIPING

- Praise is a good reward.

- If your child needs a more tangible reward, food is not a good reward because it makes him or her produce more saliva. Items such as stickers or collectibles are preferable. However, food rewards can be used for a period of time, for example, "If you can stay dry while you are watching TV then you can have a chocolate milkshake."

- Always make sure there are plenty of opportunities for success. To do this, make sure you check your child's chin when it is dry so you can give the praises he or she so deserves.

---

[1] These are called ear alarms. They are available through many Internet sources. Please see your speech–language pathologist about further information.

Getting Those Lips Together and Working

Many children have lax lips. When they are at rest, they sit open. The dribble runs over them. Some children have a retracted and short upper lip. Some children have teeth that stick out so their lips cannot meet. If your child cannot bring his or her lips together, it is more difficult to swallow properly, which may result in dribbling. Try to make these exercises fun. Sometimes you can have team games.

STRENGTHENING WEAK LIPS WITH EXERCISES

- Have fun with facial expressions, for example, smiling, frowning, pulling faces in the mirror (see Figure B.9).

- Try lip articulations: mmmm bbbb ppppp, raspberries.

- Play kissing games: put lipstick on the lips and leave a kiss on a mirror or tissue (or any part of the body), blow musical instruments, for example, harmonicas or party whistles (see Figure B.10).

- Try blowing games, such as blowing out candles (start with one candle and work up), puffing bits of tissue or table-tennis balls across the table (see Figures B.11 and B.12). You can try blowing out your cheeks and pushing the air from one side to another. Use a mirror and see if you can get the child to copy.

- Hold paper or spatulas, or something similar, between the lips. See how long the child can hold them between his or her lips.

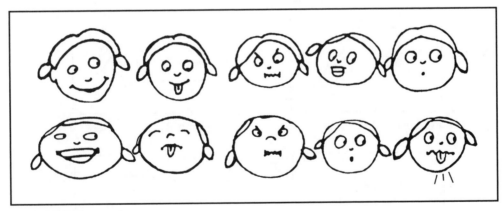

FIGURE B.9. Ten faces.

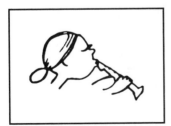

FIGURE B.10. Recorder.

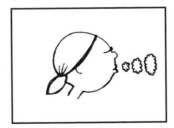

FIGURE B.11. Puff out air.

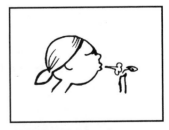

FIGURE B.12. Blow out candle.

- Suck liquid up a straw (see Figure B.13). Start with a short straw. Clear plastic tubing may be easier to use than paper straws. Thicken the liquid—for example, a thick shake—to make it more difficult.

- Play games that require sucking air up a straw to pick up a pea or bead at the end of the straw (see Figure B.14). See how many peas you can get into a container in 3 minutes.

- Use an oral screen (see Figure B.15). The screen is placed between the teeth and the lips and then pulled gently. The child tightens his or her lips onto the screen to keep it in the mouth. Pretend to be a football player! You can do the same thing with a button on a string (the button is held between the lips). You can buy ready-made oral screens from Dentaurum, Inc.[1] Some children might find it more useful to have one individually designed by a dentist. The dentist can then make changes to it to help the continuing function of the lips. This would mean making a number of trips to a dentist.

LENGTHENING THAT UPPER LIP

If your child's top lip does not move properly to meet the lower lip it may be because the muscles are tight and have shortened. We try to assist the movement of the top lip by doing the following:

- Place the flat of your finger between the nose and the top lip and press firmly.

- Use two fingers on either side of your child's nose, start from just below the bridge of the nose. Press firmly as you follow the outline of the side of the nose. When you reach the level of the nostrils, put your thumbs under the top lip and continue to pull down until your fingers meet (see Figure B.16). Sometimes you can vibrate a little with your fingers as you do it.

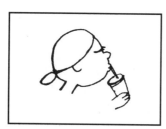

FIGURE B.13. Drink.

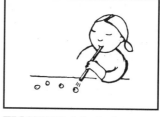

FIGURE B.14. Suck peas.

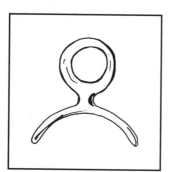

FIGURE B.15. Oral screen.

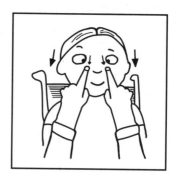

FIGURE B.16. Lengthening upper lip.

---

[1] Oral screens can be obtained from Dentaurum, Inc., 10 Pheasant Run, Newtown, PA 18940 (phone: 215/968-2858; fax: 215/968-0809; e-mail: sales@dentaurum-us.com).

- Use the oral screen. This can stimulate the top lip to move.

- Use any of the exercises mentioned in the Strengthening Weak Lips with Exercises section to help the lips come together.

INCREASING SWALLOWING

Sometimes placing the flat of your finger between your child's nose and top lip helps bring about a swallow and better lip closure (see Figure B.17).

ALTERATION OF POSTURE AND JAW CONTROL

The relationship between body and head posture, jaw control, and swallowing is complex. For children with severe physical disabilities, their wheelchair position (e.g., reclining or upright) may affect their ability to swallow and bring their lips together. Initially, full head and neck control may be required (see Figures B.18 and B.19). Children should be encouraged to take control of their own posture once they understand what they need to do.

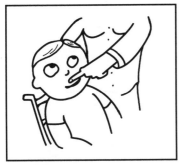

FIGURE B.17. Increasing swallowing.

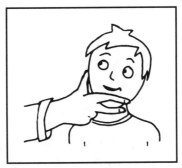

FIGURE B.18. Jaw control.

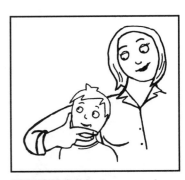

FIGURE B.19. Jaw control, with adult and child.

Keeping Up Appearances

Saliva causes staining of clothes and can be smelly and offensive. Bibs can be changed frequently, but as the child grows older there needs to be more appropriate ways of disguising the dribbling. Here are some ideas:

- Scarves may be worn around the neck to absorb the excess saliva. These may be backed with absorbent fabric such as toweling (see Figure B.20). Matching scarves worn with different outfits can be a sophisticated way to disguise the dribbling. You may need to have several of one color, because they will need to be changed regularly.

- Toweling panels can be sewn into windbreakers to absorb excess saliva. Using Kylie[1] material (a washable material used for incontinence products), you can sew a piece under a sweater so that you keep the wet fabric away from the skin.

- Vests, which can be easily changed, can be designed to go over dresses (see Figures B.21 and B.22).

- Velcro can be sewn onto clothes and motifs and collars attached (see Figure B.23). When the motif gets wet it can be quickly replaced with another one.

- Windbreakers that have a raised motif on the front can give the appearance of a drier windbreaker.

- Plain materials show the dribbling more. Choose patterned materials (see Figure B.24).

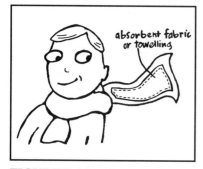

FIGURE B.20. Absorbent fabric.

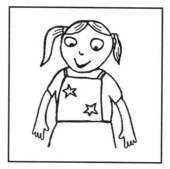

FIGURE B.21. Star vest.

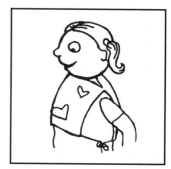

FIGURE B.22. Heart vest.

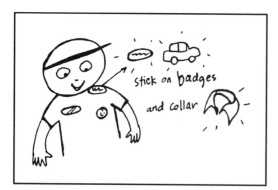

FIGURE B.23. Stick-on badges.

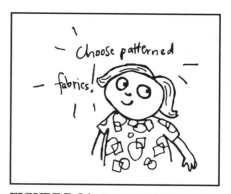

FIGURE B.24. Patterned fabric.

[1]Kylie material can be purchased from Hybrand Healthcare, P.O. Box 2799, Eastbourne, England BN22 9WA (phone: +44 0/8700 11 44 20; fax: +44 0/8700 11 44 30; Web site: www.hybrand.com).

INDEX

About the Authors

Amanda Scott, BApp Sci, PhD, has worked as a speech–language pathologist with people with progressive diseases for 20 years at Calvary Health Care, Melbourne, Australia. In addition, she is involved in the Swallowing Disorders Clinic, in conjunction with Mr. Neil Vallance, Head of the Department of Head and Neck Surgery, at Monash Medical Center, Melbourne, and works in neurosciences and with people with HIV/AIDS at the Alfred Hospital, Melbourne.

Hilary Johnson, Dip Sp Thy, MA, FSPAA, is a speech–language pathologist trained in England and now works in Australia. She has had a long-term interest in the area of complex communication needs and, in particular, saliva control. In 1990, she completed a research thesis on the measurement of drooling. In 1992, she was awarded a Winston Churchill traveling fellowship, and in 2001, she received the Ethel Temby award. Both awards have allowed her to travel and develop contacts and research ideas in the area of saliva control and augmentative communication. Currently, she is working as manager of the Communication Resource Centre part of SCOPE, Melbourne, Australia. She is a member of the Saliva Control Clinic at the Royal Children's Hospital and a member of the Saliva Interest Group.

About the Contributors

Janet Allaire, MA, is an assistant professor in the Department of Pediatrics, School of Medicine, University of Virginia. She is also a Patient Care Services Manager at the Kluge Children's Rehabilitation Center (KCRC), part of the Children's Medical Center at the university. As a speech–language pathologist by background and training, she has spent the past 28 years working with children with a broad range of disabilities at KCRC. In 1990, she cochaired the Consortium on Drooling and has been involved with sialorrhea ever since. She has worked with Dr. Carrie Brown since 1993 with the Chin Dry System and the Swallow Frequency Device.

Carrie Brown, PhD, received her PhD in 1985 in early childhood and special education and computer science. She was a teacher of students with severe emotional problems from 1971–1978. She was an adjunct professor at the University of North Texas from 1978–1984 and assistant director and then director of the Bioengineering Program, The Arc National Headquarters from 1984–1993. From 1993 to present, she has been the founder and president of Innovative Human Services, Inc., an assistive technology research and development company. For the past 6 years, her research efforts have been on the remediation, intervention, and research of saliva overflow, resulting in the Chin Dry System and Intraoral Saliva Vacuuming Appliance.

Margaret Foulsum, BAppSci, is currently working as chief speech–language pathologist at Bethlehem Health Care, Melbourne. She had 8 years prior experience working in a dental practice before graduating as a speech–language pathologist from La Trobe University, Melbourne, in 1995. She specializes in the area of progressive neurological disabilities and has a special interest in oral health, and secretion management specifically. In 2001, she developed the Oral Health Screening Tool.

Hubert Haberfellner, MD, is a general practitioner, pediatrician, and professor of Pediatrics at Children's University Hospital, Innsbruck, Austria. His special interests are facial and oral functions and dysfunctions. He is a committee member of the International Cerebral Palsy Society, the European Academy of Childhood Disability, and the Austrian Pediatrics Society.

Bruce Johnstone, MB, BS, FRACS, is a consultant plastic surgeon at the Royal Children's Hospital, Melbourne, where he is also a member of the saliva control team. In addition, he has been the head of the Reconstructive Plastic Surgery Unit at the Royal Melbourne Hospital. He has provided surgical intervention for children and adults with poor saliva control since 1987.

Bronwen Jones, BAppSci, has a degree in speech pathology and currently works as a speech–language pathologist at SCOPE (Vic) and in private practice. She graduated in 1980 from La Trobe University, Melbourne, and most of her career has focused on augmentative communication and working with people with severe and multiple disabilities.

Working with clients to help them manage their saliva problems is an important part of her daily clinical role.

Nicky Kilpatrick, BDS, PhD, FDS, RCPS, is the director of the Department of Dentistry at the Royal Children's Hospital, Melbourne, Australia. She is a pediatric dentist who trained originally in England but has worked more recently at the University of Sydney. She works predominantly with children with special needs and medical complications, and with those with clefts of the lip or palate.

James Lucas, BSc, MDSc, LDS, FRACDS, FICD, has worked in private general practice and is currently a pediatric dental specialist and deputy director of the Dental Department of the Royal Children's Hospital of Melbourne, Australia. He has been actively involved in undergraduate and postgraduate training and has lectured and conducted workshops extensively in Australia and overseas. His areas of research are growth and development, saliva, and children with dentofacial anomalies.

Susan Mathers, MB, MRCP, FRACP, is a neurologist at Bethlehem Health Care and Monash Medical Center, Melbourne, Australia. Her main interests are the neurophysiological control of sphincter mechanisms and clinical issues in the management of people with progressive neurological disabilities.

Dinah Reddihough, MD, BSc, FRACP, FAFRM, is director of Child Development and Rehabilitation at the Royal Children's Hospital in Melbourne, Australia, and is committed to the care of children with disabilities. She has a long-term interest in saliva control problems and is involved in research, teaching, and clinical activities in her efforts to improve outcomes in this area.